CW00585353

CONSTRUCTION AND GOVERNMENT

OF

LUNATIC ASYLUMS

AND

HOSPITALS FOR THE INSANE.

BY JOHN CONOLLY, M.D.

FELLOW OF THE ROYAL COLLEGE OF PHYSICIANS OF LONDON, AND
PHYSICIAN TO THE MIDDLESEX LUNATIC ASYLUM AT HANWELL.

WITH PLANS.

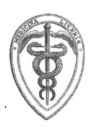

LONDON:
JOHN CHURCHILL, PRINCES STREET, SOHO.
MDCCCXLVII.

C. AND J. ADLARD, PRINTERS, BARTHOLOMEW CLOSE.

The greater part of the following pages is a reprint from Lectures published in the Lancet, in 1846, supplementary to a Clinical Course on the Symptoms and Treatment of the various forms of Insanity.

HANWELL, *March*, 1847.

CONTENTS.

PAGE

CHAPTER I. Want of additional County Lunatic Asylums for the Curable and Incurable.—Site and general Plan best suited to an Asylum; Errors of existing Plans.—Arrangement of Galleries and Sleeping Rooms; and for the Classification of the Patients.—Inconveniences of large Dormitories 1

CHAPTER II. Arrangement of Galleries and Sleeping Rooms.—Inspection-plates.—Doors and Windows.—Warming and Ventilation,—Lighting at Night.—Cleanliness.—Sources of Offensive Smells.—Dormitories, Water-closets, Sinks, &c. &c., their most convenient Arrangement.— Store-rooms. — Washing-rooms. — Baths. — Modifications required in Asylums for Patients of various Classes . . 26

CHAPTER III. Situation of Wards for the Elderly and Feeble.—Infirmaries.—Former Abuses of Restraints in Wards for the Sick.—Present Arrangements.—Airing Courts and Grounds.—Classification out of doors.—Recreations without and within doors.—Evening Entertainments.—Clothing of the Insane 45

CHAPTER IV. Diet of the Insane.—Its Influence on Recoveries, and on the Mortality of Asylums.—Hanwell Dietary.—Average weekly Cost of each Patient.—Employment of the Insane: its use and abuse . 65

PAGE

CHAPTER V. Attendants, Appointment and Qualifications of.—Their daily Duties.—Arrangements for Night-watching in an Asylum . 83

CHAPTER VI. General Duties of Attendants in Asylums.—Their proper Government.—Peculiar Duties of Attendants on Private Patients . 105

CHAPTER VII. Concluding Chapter.—Religious Services in an Asylum. —Schools.—Government of Asylums.—Treatment of Officers.— Position and Duties of the Medical Superintendent . . . 122

APPENDIX. Cost of Building Asylums 145
Statistics 146
Incurable Patients 154
Schools for the Insane and the Idiotic at the Salpêtrière and Bicêtre Asylums, Paris 156
Abolition of Personal Coercion 163
Religious Services in Asylums 177
Effects of the separation of Patients, supposed to be incurable, from the curable Patients 178
Plans of Asylums 181

CONSTRUCTION AND GOVERNMENT

OF

LUNATIC ASYLUMS.

CHAPTER I.

*Want of additional County Lunatic Asylums for the Curable and Incurable.
—Site and general Plan best suited to an Asylum; Errors of existing
Plans.—Arrangement of Galleries and Sleeping Rooms; and for the
Classification of the Patients.—Inconveniences of large Dormitories.*

THE construction, arrangement, and government of Asylums
for the Insane are subjects at this time so important, in consequence of the many new asylums about to be built in
England and Wales, and in Ireland, as well to deserve very careful consideration. Like everything connected with such institutions, they are of consequence in relation to the treatment
of the patients; to their bodily as well as to their mental
health; to their comfort or to their recovery. In offering
some observations on these subjects, the result of my experience as a Physician for some years resident in one of the
largest asylums in the world, I would first remark, that a
lunatic asylum is intended to be not merely a place of security
but a place of cure; and that every case of insanity is curable or
improvable up to a certain point. The recovery of the curable,
the improvement of the incurable, the comfort and happiness

1

of all the patients, should therefore steadily be kept in view by the architect from the moment in which he commences his plan; and should be the no less constant guide of the governing bodies of asylums in every law and regulation which they make, and every resolution to which they come.

By a recent Act of Parliament (8th and 9th Vict. cap. 126, August 8, 1845), it is directed that asylums shall be provided for the pauper lunatics of every county and borough in England and Wales. The total number of insane poor in England and Wales has been stated to be about 17,000. (*Report of Metropolitan Commissioners in Lunacy,* 1844.) Of these not more than about 4500 are yet provided for in asylums; and in each county having no asylum it has become an object of solicitude, with those who are to furnish the funds for establishing asylums, to make such provision in a manner as little burthensome as possible. The magistrates appear to be everywhere anxious to comply with the spirit of the Act, of which the general tendency is to improve the condition of those who are insane and destitute of resources. But considerable opposition has arisen in several counties to any proposals for erecting a county asylum; and this opposition has been supported in some cases by an assertion that pauper lunatics are not only more cheaply provided for in private licensed houses than in county asylums, but that the number of cures effected in the private houses is greater. In some counties or parts of counties, also, a preference is shown for the plan of attaching small asylums to the workhouses instead of building one large asylum for the whole county; and this arrangement is sanctioned by the Act. Each of these methods of providing for pauper lunatics is very objectionable.

In preferring either private licensed houses, or small asylums, or lunatic wards attached to workhouses, to asylums especially adapted to the insane, the state of those to be provided for is entirely disregarded, and the actual condition of pauper lunatics, both in workhouses and in private licensed houses is entirely overlooked. The insane poor are of necessity exposed in both such places to innumerable disadvantages, only to be avoided in larger public asylums. Their diet, their clothing, their lodging, are all generally of the most wretched description; the means of occupation are very limited; space for exercise is wanting; means of recreation and amusement are unthought of or unknown; and security is only effected by confining the limbs of the violent or troublesome, or by buildings so contrived as almost to shut out light and air, and utterly to exclude cheerfulness. All these circumstances are manifestly unfavorable to the recovery, or even to the amendment of those thus confined; and, whilst there is not any foundation for the assertion, that the number of cures, in curable or recent cases, is greater in private licensed houses for paupers than in public asylums, the mortality in such licensed houses has been shown far to exceed that of the public institutions.

Of the recent cases sent into public asylums, if not epileptic or affected with paralysis, about fifty per cent. recover: this appears to be the real average of recoveries in all public asylums, calculating the recoveries on the average daily number of patients in them; and it probably represents the actual curability of insanity, exclusive of relapses. But at present the public or county asylums are nearly filled with old and incurable cases; the patients having been first sent, in the recent and curable state of their malady, to the private licensed houses, or detained in workhouses, and only transferred to the county asylums when they became unmanageable or were considered to be incurable.

As regards the question of expense, also, it appears that when once a county asylum is built and opened the patients are maintained in it at less cost than in private licensed houses; the average charge per week in the licensed houses being 8s. 11½d.; and the average cost in county asylums 7s. 6¼d.; constituting a saving to the parishes of nearly 1s. 6d. per week for each patient; which in an asylum for 300 patients would constitute a considerable annual saving to the rate-payers of the county. How much better the pauper lunatic is taken care of in any

well-conducted county asylum is easily to be ascertained by
inspection.

According to the Act of Parliament already alluded to, all
plans for the contemplated asylums must be submitted to the
Commissioners in Lunacy for their approval. It most unfortunately happens that the Commissioners have adopted an
opinion that it is practicable and safe to provide for chronic
cases, or for incurable lunatics, at much less expense than
for recent and curable cases. "The great expenses," they say,
"of a lunatic hospital are unnecessary for incurable patients :
the medical staff, the number of attendants, the minute classification, and the other requisites of an hospital for the cure of
disease, are not required to the same extent. An establishment,
therefore, upon a much less expensive scale would be sufficient." (*Report*, p. 92.)

This conclusion may at first sight appear reasonable to
those not familiar with the insane ; but I believe that by all
who have lived in asylums it will be pronounced to be fallacious, and not unattended with danger. The views of the
Commissioners in this and other respects have already led to
the suspension of what appeared to me to be the best plans
ever proposed for asylums ; and will, I fear, lead to the com-
mitting of great errors in several which are in preparation.
These consequences, and the sanction given to attach lunatic
asylums to workhouses, will go far to undo the good which
has been slowly and with much difficulty effected since the
Parliamentary Inquiry into the state of asylums in 1815.

Not to dwell on the impracticability of the absolute division
of the incurable from the curable patients in any asylum ; or
on the cruelty of condemning the incurable to what would
appear to them to be a hopeless prison ; or on the possibility of sometimes including curable patients in this condem-
nation—I cannot but remark, that, in expressing the opinion
which I have quoted, the Commissioners in Lunacy seem to
have forgotten that a large proportion of the incurable among
the insane are even more sensible to all surrounding circum-

stances than the curable who are labouring under a recent attack; that the whole character of the life of such incurable patients depends on the manner in which they are treated and taken care of; that some of them well know the asylum to be their permanent home; and that most of them, so far from requiring fewer, actually require more means of occupation, more space for exercise, greater opportunities of recreation than the curable, and a greater variety of comfortable arrangements to reconcile them to their situation, and to maintain that habitual content and tranquillity which distinguish a well-regulated asylum from a miserable madhouse.

It must also have been entirely forgotten, that many of the incurable are paralysed and feeble, yet occasionally delirious; that many are epileptic, and occasionally furious; and that among those who are neither paralysed nor epileptic, and who are generally tranquil and inoffensive, many are yet liable, several times in every year, to attacks of recurrent mania or melancholia, of which the symptoms do not differ in any respect from those in recent and curable cases, and render all the requirements of treatment, and all provisions for superintendence, and all precautions for safety, as indispensable as in an asylum containing recent and curable cases alone.

The observations made at page 100 of the Report already cited, relative to the necessity of exercise and occupation, and of the services of experienced attendants, even for harmless and incurable lunatics, seem indeed to admit a necessity so positively denied in the same Report, at page 92. But it is greatly to be feared, that an opinion which comes recommended by a promise of saving much in the expense of providing for pauper lunatics, will be too readily and generally adopted.

Lastly, and more than all, it seems to be forgotten by those who altogether object to County Lunatic Asylums, on account of their expense, either for the incurable or the curable among the insane poor, that those afflicted persons have the double claim upon society arising from poverty and from malady; and that the benevolent consideration so cheerfully given, in all Christian countries, to the sick poor who are not insane, ought at least to be as freely extended to those labouring under sickness and infirmity of mind; many of whom, if placed in circumstances favorable to recovery, may be restored to mental health and to usefulness; and all of whom may be improved to a certain extent by proper care.

As it is scarcely possible to construct a building intended for the residence of several hundreds of human beings, in a state of unsound mind, without finding that some inconveniences are inherent in its design, a new plan is at present generally adopted whenever a new asylum is built, and, generally, some new inconveniences are incurred. In building and in governing asylums it is just the same, and partly from the same cause; a dislike to appeal to the authority of medical men who have lived in asylums, and among the insane, and who alone know what the insane require. So no two plans are alike, and almost all asylums are under regulations, several of which are injudicious, often interfering with the comfort of the officers, and sometimes directly impeding the improvement of the patients.

There are scarcely any works written expressly on this subject with which the English reader is familiar, or to which he can safely be referred. Several sound observations concerning the plan of asylums are, however, scattered through the writings of M. Esquirol; and many valuable remarks are contained in Sir Wm. Ellis's work on Insanity. A work, by the celebrated Dr. Jacobi, of Siegburg, entirely devoted to the construction and management of asylums, has also been translated into English by Mr. Kitching, under the superintendence of Mr. Tuke, of York, who, although not a medical man, is known all over the world as one of the most enlightened friends of the insane. Mr. Tuke has contributed to the translation a valuable preface, and notes. Dr. Jacobi's work contains a great number of useful suggestions; but the reader should be cautioned that they were written thirteen years ago, and are all conformable to the old system of restraint and force, although tempered by the author's evident kindness of heart and good understanding.

In most of the old asylums the architects appear to have had regard solely to the safe keeping of the inmates, and the buildings resemble prisons rather than hospitals for the cure of insanity. Even now, high and gloomy walls, narrow or inaccessible windows, heavy and immovable tables and benches, and prison regulations applied to the officers and attendants, attest the prevalence of mistaken and limited views. It appears to me, that not only should no general plan of a lunatic asylum be determined upon without being submitted to the consideration of a physician acquainted with the character, habits, and wants of the insane, but that no alteration should be made in an asylum without a reference to its resident medical officers. They alone at once see, or at least appear much to regard, the effects of rash and unadvised modifications. The building of a wall, the raising of a roof, the alteration of a door or window, or window-shutter, may materially affect the daily comfort of numerous patients, and the safety of others. What an anxiety for mere safety has suggested, may at once be seen by them to be inconsistent with light and cheerfulness, and apparent conveniences will to them always appear objectionable if purchased by a diminution of proper ventilation and warmth.

The only way to avoid the defects apparent in so many existing asylums, without incurring new ones, would be to take a careful preparatory survey of the character and requirements of the insane, so that a just estimate might be formed of what is generally desirable, and what is wanted in particular portions of the building only. To render this survey effective, the aid of medical men who have lived in asylums should be required at every step.

Although the first thing demanded by society, when we undertake to relieve it of the presence of those who cannot be at large consistently with the safety of themselves or others, is their perfect security, it must be remembered that this security does not require gloom, or a frightful apparatus. We require that the building should be on a healthy site, freely admitting light and air, and drainage. Space should be allowed for summer and winter exercise, for various employments, and for all the purposes of domestic economy. Warmth must be provided for during the winter, light for the winter evenings, coolness and shade in the summer. Separate wards and bed-rooms for the tranquil, for the sick, for the helpless, for the noisy, the unruly, or violent, and the dirty; a supply of water so copious, and a drainage so complete, that the baths, water-closets, and building in general, may always be kept perfectly clean and free from bad odours. There should be workshops and workrooms, and schoolrooms, separate from the wards, and cheerfully situated; a chapel, conveniently accessible from both sides of the asylum; as also a kitchen, a laundry, a bakehouse, a brewhouse, and rooms for stores, and all the requisites for gardening and farming; and also a surgery, and all that is necessary for the medical staff. All these are indispensable in every large public asylum.

There can be no doubt that the best site for an asylum is a gentle eminence, of which the soil is naturally dry, and in a fertile and agreeable country, near enough to high roads, a railway, or a canal, and a town, to facilitate the supply of stores, and the occasional visits of the friends of the patients, and to diversify the scene without occasioning disturbance. A very elevated situation is often attended with the disadvantage of a deficient supply of water, and a difficulty in adding to the extent of the building. An extremely exposed and cold situation should be avoided; for if lunatics do not complain, they are still injured by severe cold. The circulation is generally feeble in the insane, and coldness of the extremities is usual with them. Consumption is very frequent in asylums; and the paralysed patients, who are generally numerous, suffer serious aggravations of their malady in the cold weather of winter. Mr. Tuke justly points out the ineligibility, in this climate, of a site level with a running stream; and observes, that a moderate elevation does not necessarily induce the evils of exposure and publicity, as supposed by Jacobi.

Patients of all classes derive advantage from the circumstances of situation just mentioned; and if it is intended to receive patients of the educated classes into the house, it should unquestionably be situated amidst scenery calculated to give pleasure to such persons when of sane mind. Those whose faculties have never been cultivated derive little satisfaction from the loveliest aspects of nature, and experience little emotion amidst the grandest. The sun rises and sets, the stars shine and fall, the hills reflect all the variety of brightness and shadow, of wildness and of verdure, and yet are scarcely noticed with more than mere passing attention. But when education has called the higher faculties into life, impressions upon them, even from external nature, become powerful for good or ill, and in the case of a mind diseased, may act as remedies, or aggravate the malady. The celebrated Robert Hall attributed much of his unhappy state of mind, and even his temporary insanity, to a change of residence from a picturesque and interesting part of the country to a cheerless plain, of which the dulness, flatness, and invariable monotony saddened his heart. Cowper, whose writings indicate exquisite sympathy with the sights and sounds of common rural retirement, and who, like Robert Hall, was occasionally afflicted with insanity, felt awe-struck and overwhelmed when visiting a friend whose house was situated among lofty hills covered with trees. There are few persons of any degree of education much of whose daily and habitual pleasure does not arise from the view of the objects around them; and the first desire of all who can quit the crowd and toil of business, is to be where they can enjoy " a prospect," or to surround their houses with shrubs and flowers. Even in the populous city, the pent-up artisan has a bird, to sing to him whilst he works, and a few flowers, which he cultivates with care. We must not neglect such instincts and capacities if we profess to cure

1 §

diseased minds. Our practice can only securely rest on the consideration of everything, great or little, capable of affecting the mind beneficially or hurtfully.

The more experience I have of the duties to be performed in a lunatic asylum, the more strongly I become impressed with the inconveniences attending any part of the building consisting of more than two stories. The third story is difficult of access and egress for the patients; it is unavoidably dull, and it becomes almost unavoidably neglected. It is equally opposed to good classification and to proper superintendence; and it causes too many insane persons to be included in the same extent of ground, rendering ventilation more difficult, and decreasing the healthiness of the establishment. There should be no inhabited attics; no bedrooms or dormitories in the basement of the building. All the rooms should be above ground, so as easily to be visited, and to make it easy for the patients to go out of doors. Wide and easy stone staircases, with square landing-places, and without acute-angled steps, should connect the upper and the lower story. Light and air should pervade every part of the building; water and warmth should be everywhere equally supplied.

It is particularly necessary to observe, that almost every desirable quality, both in the construction and government of an asylum, becomes more difficult to be obtained or preserved when the size of the asylum is greater than is required for 360 or 400 patients. This preliminary observation will apply to all the suggestions I shall have to make. In an asylum of a larger size, the architect must sacrifice much to expediency, and the government of the establishment can scarcely preserve any uniformity of character.

A great fault is generally committed in the original construction of county asylums, which subsequently entails many other faults. The asylum is usually erected merely for the supposed actual number of lunatics within a county; and, in consequence of the incurable patients not being discharged, the building becomes, in the course of ten years, crowded with nearly double the number first provided for. Provision is made for these, first by means of the erection or extension of wings, to which, if the original plan has been well devised, there exists no objection; but afterward, by piling a third story wherever it can be raised, or by excavating rooms and wards under ground. These arrangements have all the disadvantages which I have mentioned. They render proper classification, either within doors or without, almost impossible, and the preservation of order difficult. By the accumulation of so many persons, day and night, in a lofty building, many of whom can seldom leave the wards, and no one of whom is in perfect health, the asylum becomes subject to every atmospheric and terrestrial influence unfavorable to life. If no epidemic outbreak alarms the governors into an investigation and reform of buildings so arranged, or ill-placed, or otherwise unhealthy, the inmates are merely all brought to a low standard of health; to uneasiness, suffering, and a disposition to illness. There is always a risk of more active disease; and this may not only depopulate the institution to a great extent, but spread pestilence around it. Lessons of this kind are learnt with unwillingness, because they are opposed to the strong avarice which vitiates all social provision for the poor; and they are also soon forgotten. The terrible examples afforded in 1832, when the malignant cholera last visited us, are so unheeded, that when the malady comes again, it will find almost every asylum, public and private, equally unprepared with reasonable preservatives against it.

The Derbyshire magistrates, finding that the number of insane paupers in their county at this time amounts to 216, have designed an asylum capable of holding 360, so that no addition to the building may be required for some time; and I regret to learn that this wise provision has constituted one of the objections made to it by the Commissioners. The Hanwell Asylum was opened in 1831, for 300 patients; it now con-

tains about 1000; and another asylum is already required in
the county for nearly as many more.

Among the various forms of asylums adopted by architects,
I believe there is none so convenient as one in which the main
part of the building is in one line; the residence of the chief
physician or other officers being in the centre, and also a
chapel, and a large square room in which the patients may be
occasionally assembled from either side of the asylum on the
occasion of an evening entertainment, and which may also be
capable of division for schools; the kitchen, laundry, workshops, and various offices, being arranged behind these central
buildings. To this main line, wings of moderate extent being
added at right angles in each direction, the building assumes
what is called the H form; but it is desirable that the length
of front should be more extended than that of the wings; and
it is better still if the wings only extend in one direction, and
away from the front, or northward, supposing the front of the
asylum to be to the south. At Hanwell the wings advance
from the main front at right angles in one direction only, and
new wings have been added at right angles with the first,
in the same direction as the main front. It is evident that a
building of this shape, long and narrow, consisting of a succession of galleries or corridors, with bedrooms on one side
only, may be moderately perflated by every wind that blows—
an advantage extremely salutary to those who pass their whole
time in it. The want of proper ventilation is chiefly incidental to the angles of the building, and to the centre, and
should be carefully provided against. In hot climates, exposure to the sun is a frequent cause of cerebral excitement,
and many of our patients persist in exposing their bare heads
to the sun in the hottest weather, until it is scarcely possible
to touch their heads with one's hand. But in this country the
hot season is of short duration, and it is especially necessary
to consider that no gallery within the house, and no airing-
ground exterior to it, should be deprived of some share of sun-

shine in the winter, as well as of free access of air, and some shade in summer. Quadrangular buildings, (unless the quadrangle is very large, and the buildings are very low,) and circular buildings, and central towers or crescents with radiating wings in three or more directions, are open to great objections on every account. A north and south aspect is perhaps as convenient as any other, and the galleries and day-rooms should certainly face the south, or south-east. If the houses of the officers are also to the south, and the kitchen and other offices behind the centre, the principal approach to the asylum must be on the south likewise, and being exposed to the windows of all the galleries and day-rooms, should be screened by an avenue or a semicircular plantation of trees or shrubs. If the central house projects a little from the main front, and has the kitchen, &c., behind it, the projection and the approach will form a complete division between the east and west galleries, and the male and female patients will be effectually separated, both in the front and at the back of the asylum, those of one sex being out of sight of those of the other, both in the galleries and airing-courts.

Much ornament or decoration, external or internal, is useless, and rather offends irritable patients than gives any satisfaction to the more contented. In some of the Italian asylums, busts, pictures, and ornaments abound, and the walls are painted with figures representing various allegories or histories. These would appear more likely to rouse morbid associations than to do any good. I also disapprove of painting numbers and titles on the walls of airing-courts, by which the walls are disfigured, and the patients are reminded of their confinement as insane persons when walking out for relaxation, or led to consider themselves prisoners. The wards and bedrooms also should only be designated by simple numbers.

When it is remembered that many patients are sent to an asylum whose senses are as perfect, and whose feelings are as acute, as those of sane people, and that from the moment they enter the outer gate everything becomes remedial with them, or the reverse, the reason will at once be seen why the external aspect of an asylum should be more cheerful than imposing, more resembling a well-built hospital than a place of seclusion or imprisonment. It should be surrounded by gardens, or a farm. Even the part of the building to which the patient is first admitted is important. In the new asylum about to be built in the county of Middlesex, I feel sure that the magistrates will anxiously avoid an inconvenience which is very much felt in the present building, where the reception rooms open directly into large towers, in which a circular staircase is so guarded with iron palisades as to give the patients looking through them, in the three different stories, the appearance of persons shut up in tiers of iron cages. A very painful impression is often made by this prospect being suddenly presented to the new comer; and it is strongest in those in whom the hope of recovery renders the avoidance of all counteracting agencies of the most consequence. The reception-room should be a cheerful and neatly-furnished sitting-room, and so situated that the newly-admitted patients can proceed from it to whatever part of the asylum it is thought best they should be sent. Thus, violent and noisy patients would not be led shouting and struggling through tranquil wards; and timid and quiet patients would not have to pass along corridors containing patients whose unfamiliar looks agitate or affright them.

In all building arrangements for the insane, a very liberal space should be allowed. The galleries should be spacious, and the doors wide, particularly those through which a crowd of patients must often pass. The same rule should be observed in the kitchens, laundry, store-rooms, &c., of which, in many respects, the Hanwell Asylum presents an excellent example. The galleries at Hanwell are, however, only ten feet wide; those of Bethlem are much wider. The galleries in the Kent Asylum are fourteen feet wide, and those at Siegburg twenty feet. A width of twelve feet, with a height of eleven, seems to be suitable for the galleries of a county asylum. A public asylum is ordinarily a series of galleries, out of which almost all the bedrooms open on one side, whilst on the other large windows and doors open on the airing-courts and gardens; and this seems to be, upon the whole, a convenient arrangement, as some patients like occasionally to go into their rooms for the sake of quiet; and others who require seclusion are thus not removed from occasional notice and convenient superintendence. The galleries should be light and cheerful; several small tables and chairs, or fixed seats, should be placed between the windows; the windows should be low and large, affording a view of pleasant courts and shrubberies. Those in the galleries at Hanwell are two feet six inches from the floor; the dimensions of each window being six feet six inches by three feet six inches. It is desirable to have plants in the windows, and here and there birdcages; and the windows most exposed to the sun should be provided with green blinds. The part of the building which is in one line cannot well be prolonged further on each side of the centre building than to form two galleries on each story, on each side, each gallery having as many sleeping-rooms opening from it as are required for twenty-five or thirty patients; as many as can, without disadvantage, be placed together in one ward, under two attendants. Even to accommodate this number in each ward,—two-thirds having single rooms,—it becomes necessary to have rooms on both sides, which is not desirable. As there must be a communication from the gallery nearest the centre to the next gallery, the first has usually the inconvenience of being without any end window. This has been avoided in the plan for the Derby Asylum, already referred to, by causing the second ward to be placed sufficiently withdrawn from the first to leave a space for a gallery window. This occasions no kind of deformity in the building, and is productive of very obvious advantage. The same principle may be preserved at the angles where the wings commence; and the difference between a gallery with a window at the end and one ending with a wall or a door is very great. This plan

would afford two wards on each story, on each side of the
centre, constituting the main line; or eight wards, each containing thirty patients; thus providing for 240 patients. For
this an extended frontage is necessary, which it may not always
be easy to command, but which should always be provided for,
if possible, when constructing a large asylum. Each wing
would contain one ward for thirty patients on each floor, or
four wards capable of receiving 120 patients; the whole number of patients being then 360. Small T ends at the extremity of the wings might accommodate twenty more patients
on each side, making 400. All the arrangements are easy
up to this point; but the moment it is passed difficulties
commence.

With spacious, well-lighted, cheerful galleries, of which the
floors are boarded, I have long been of opinion that what are
called dayrooms can scarcely be required, except as an additional means of comfort, in wards appropriated to the convalescent, and those for whom greater tranquillity is required
from the time of admission, or by whom it is beginning to be
appreciated. But even for these, a separate room, where
opportunities of reading and writing, or hearing music, are
afforded to a few at a time, is far better. So, also, for the
wards in which most of the patients are capable of being
employed, it is better to have workrooms detached a little
from the wards. The change is agreeable and salutary to the
patients, and they may still be under efficient superintendence. But the galleries may be made a kind of sitting-
room for such patients as prefer remaining in it, by means of
a few work-tables, or reading-tables, or chairs. Some of the
female patients, and a few of the male patients will always
be found to employ themselves most comfortably in their own
bedrooms; and this should be permitted in certain cases.

At Hanwell, or in any other asylum where the wards have
a dayroom branching off at an angle from the gallery, proper
superintendence must always be difficult. If anything happens in the gallery, the excuse is, that the attendant was in

the dayroom; and if anything happens in the dayroom, that the attendant was in the gallery: and although no ward ought to have fewer than two attendants, one of them must often be absent. In the wards for the most refractory of the Hanwell patients, there are no dayrooms: as the galleries are not wider in that part of the building than nine feet, and have rooms on both sides, recesses with windows are substituted for dayrooms, and also one end of the gallery in two of them; and when you enter one of these wards, you can generally see all the patients and both the attendants. In the quieter wards, you may often walk from one end of the gallery to another without seeing any attendant, which is always inconvenient, and sometimes unsafe. In the plan for the Derby Asylum, the wide galleries have a deep bay, equi-distant from both ends, well lighted, and opposite to a fireplace; and by this plan every advantage is secured, including that constant superintendence which is indispensable to preserving order and comfort, and without which the prevention of mischief—which is an important element of the non-restraint treatment—is quite impracticable.

If there are no dayrooms, the patients dine at tables in the recesses, and occasionally work there if they please; other tables may be placed along the walls, letting down when not wanted. Troublesome patients are even more conveniently watched and attended to at dinner time at these tables; they do not sit opposite to other patients; they can easily be removed from the table if necessary, and always be efficiently overlooked by the attendants standing behind them. Our galleries at Hanwell have stone floors, which I believe the committee, as well as the medical officers, would gladly exchange for oak boards, but that the alteration would now be attended with much trouble and expense. The stone floors are the cause of many bruises to the epileptic, and sometimes to the paralytic and feeble; and in the winter they seem rapidly to abstract all the caloric from the lower extremities—an inconvenience felt both by the patients and their attendants.

No inconvenience arises from the walls of the galleries being unwainscoted; they are usually painted of a light-brown colour to the height of four or five feet, with a deeper-brown border, and the upper part of the wall and the ceiling are whitewashed. An appearance of cleanliness was formerly given to the floors of the galleries and bedrooms, by having them daily rubbed with soft stone; but the dust or white powder thence arising pervaded everything, and the practice is now discontinued.

The Hanwell Asylum is a succession of such galleries, and on each side, in the galleries nearest to the central tower, we have the most tranquil patients, and some of the newly-admitted, and some of the convalescent. At the end of the main line of the building, where the first wings commence, we have, on each side, an infirmary. The first wings are appropriated, on the female side, to the epileptic, imbecile, loquacious, and troublesome; and on the male side, to the orderly, and the more rational of the epileptics, the more imbecile male patients being in a basement ward in the second wing. The towers, at which the first wings end and the second commence, contain wards for clean and industrious patients; and the second wings, being remotest from the centre, are assigned to the noisy, the refractory, and the dirty. The patients are so arranged, that the tranquil are separated from those only moderately or occasionally tranquil, and all these from the very noisy and dirty; and these general divisions will be found necessary in every public asylum.

How much the mere plan of the building has to do with the arrangement of the patients, will be understood after very little reflection on the consequences of having each ward made a passage to the next, from the centre of the building to the extremities. Some of the patients at the very extremities come to the central chapel, and in doing so, traverse every ward on the same floor: they must come through some of the wards every day for the dinners of their ward, or to the laundry, or to the storeroom; and if all these are situated in the centre of the building, there must be a frequent and confused intermingling of the patients of all classes and descriptions. All this, however, is avoided in the Derby plan, by means of a corridor on the outside of the building, running beneath the windows of the sleeping-rooms; and such a corridor is practicable on both stories; to this, however, the Commissioners have made the reasonable objection, that as the windows of the bedrooms must be above such corridors, they will be improperly high. Means may perhaps be found to obviate this inconvenient result; and, certainly, the corridor on the upper story may be dispensed with.

But, whatever arrangements are made, the more precise and formal classification laid down in some works on insanity is impracticable. The state of bodily health of some of the patients, the particular occupation to which they are attached, their partialities and dislikes for or of particular parts of the asylum, or particular patients, must often be taken into consideration. It is remarkable that Dr. Jacobi, who lays down rules for such a minute classification of patients as I should myself not attempt to enforce, is strongly averse to the separation of the convalescents even from the worst of the patients. He derides it as the humane idea of theorists. I believe the absolute separation of the curable from the incurable neither to be practicable nor desirable; and I know that the incurable patients are generally better companions for the curable than other curable patients are; but certainly the convalescent should be guarded from the society of the more agitated and turbulent patients; indeed, they usually petition for removal to a quiet ward, or for occupation out of the wards; and in a large asylum, with large wards, it is scarcely possible to have one ward which is perfectly free from occasional disturbance. A minuter subdivision of the patients would obviate this, but a greater number of attendants would then become necessary.

I cannot anywhere more appropriately express my opinion that every asylum should be fire-proof, than now, when speak-

ing of the arrangement of the galleries. As it is necessary to
lock the door of every patient's bedroom at night, and as each
window is secured, the window-frames being of cast-iron, the
escape of the patients in case of fire would entirely depend
on the attendants being able to go through every gallery, and
unlock every bedroom door. To do this, the doors being at
least twenty in number in each gallery, and steadily to direct
the patients along the galleries to the proper door or staircase
of escape, every window being too strongly secured to permit
egress—would only be a possible duty with the consciousness
of the general safety of the rooms, the floors, and the roof.
To do it with fire blazing about them, or thick smoke filling
the galleries, amidst all the confusion which a fire in an asylum creates among sane people, and the additional and frightful confusion to be expected among the patients, would be so
extremely difficult, that its performance could not reasonably
be calculated upon. In whatever part of the building a door
was forgotten, or left locked, or in whatever gallery a patient
lingered and was overlooked, the patient must be suffocated
or burnt. The saving to be effected by omitting the simple
precaution of having all parts of the building fire-proof, is
not to be put in competition with this horrible danger.

It may generally be observed, when a patient is first admitted into an asylum, and is in a state to pay much attention
to surrounding circumstances, that the kind of sleeping-room
allotted to him becomes a source of satisfaction or of discontent. Every one who has any personal experience of sickness
and bad nights, must know how sleep is conciliated or repelled
by the temperature, the tranquillity, and even the general
aspect of the bedroom, and the appearance or quality of the
bedding and bedclothes. These feelings must be remembered
when we have to make night and day arrangements for
nervous or insane persons accustomed to the comforts of life,
and there is no necessity for forgetting them even in an asylum for the poorest lunatics. A clean and cheerful sleeping-
room, clean bedding, and a little coir matting on the stone

floor, are appreciated by the patient, and help to reconcile him to the house. We possess, indeed, in county asylums, this advantage, that our simplest accommodations and our scrupulous cleanliness constitute comforts rather above those enjoyed by the greater number of our poor patients in their sane state.

In the wards for quiet patients it is not at all necessary that the windows of the bedrooms should be so small, or so high from the floor, as they are in general in the Hanwell Asylum and many other asylums, or as they must be in wards for the refractory or very noisy. The superior cheerfulness of those bedrooms in which there are large windows is very observable at Hanwell. A window four feet six inches from the floor, and about three feet wide, would give much cheerfulness to the single-bedded rooms occupied by our quiet patients in the wards nearest to the centre tower, of which the general dimensions are eight feet six inches, by six feet eight inches, the height of the room being eleven feet six inches. Excepting in the bedrooms of wards assigned to the cleanest and quietest patients, I should not recommend boarded floors, which certainly have a tendency to retain bad smells. Brick floors become uneven, and are then inconvenient. The square Suffolk tile, laid in composition, so as to be perfectly level, has a very neat appearance, and seems to be tolerably durable. Asphalte, mastich, and other materials, have been tried in different asylums, but have not, I believe, obtained any general preference.. Whatever the material of the floor is, it should be level, and should not absorb and retain moisture. Sloping floors are mere contrivances to avoid the trouble required to preserve cleanliness or dryness, and are never necessary either in bedrooms or galleries, where the patients are properly attended to. The walls, if not plastered, may be painted or coloured to a certain height, like the galleries, the upper part of the wall and the ceiling being whitewashed. No kind of privy should be placed in any bedroom in asylums, nor any fixed urinal, nor chamber utensils made of metal: it is impossible to prevent their becoming offensive. Moveable, air-tight, pierced chairs may occasionally be placed in the rooms of the sick and infirm. If everything of this kind is excluded from the bedrooms except in such cases, all the single-bedded rooms may easily be kept well ventilated by means of a circular portion of the window being made to turn so as to leave open spaces for the admission of air, and by keeping the door of the bedroom open during the day. All elaborate methods of regulating the supply of air or warmth, if requiring observance by the attendants, are objectionable, because almost sure to be neglected. If they have to bring steps in order to open and shut window-shutters and ventilators, or gratings to admit warm air, the opening and shutting will seldom be attended to. The subject of warming and ventilating will, however, be afterward spoken of.

The furniture of the bedrooms should be simple. A light cast-iron bedstead, without curtains, except in particular instances, is the best for all the quiet and orderly patients, and it is quite unnecessary to fasten it to the floor. I prefer such as are made on a simple plan, without hinges or complications of any kind. A little carpet, or a coir matting, a chair or a small bench, are things required in every room; and many patients require the further indulgence of a washing-stand, a box, a little looking-glass, and a small chest of drawers; and it is to be remembered that these become most necessary for many of the incurable patients, for whom the asylum is the only home.

Epileptic patients, and old and feeble patients, are safest in the old-fashioned crib bedstead made of deal, and varying in depth from six to twelve inches, and very little raised from the floor, the bottom being lined with lead, grooved and sloping to a central aperture; the latter arrangements being required for what are called wet or dirty patients. By means of canvas stretched on a wooden frame, made to fit the bedsteads, we avoid the necessity of straw mattresses under the coir-bed of the clean patients, and also the necessity for having any loose straw-beds for the wet and dirty, as the blankets and sheets, without a coir bed, can be placed on the canvas stretcher, two of such stretchers being assigned to each bedstead, so that one may always be ready for use, and changed for the other daily, or as often as required.

Various descriptions of beds are required for the sick, the very feeble and sinking, and the aged. To many, a feather-bed is a most desirable comfort; and an air-bed or water-bed is best adapted to cases where the skin is tender or ulcerated. Some soft pillows, of various sizes, should always be kept in the store-rooms for occasional use, and the ordinary pillows should be large, so as to raise the head; and in epileptic cases or those in which a tendency to apoplexy exists, a pillow shaped like a writing-desk, by which both the head and shoulders are well supported, is still better. In the wards for refractory and dirty patients, other arrangements become necessary. The bedsteads were formerly often employed to blockade the inside of the door, and a patient would keep everybody out, and remain silent and obstinate in the bed-room, or would threaten great violence to any one opening the door. Such a circumstance is now of very rare occurrence; but it may be prevented by having all the doors in the refractory wards made to open outwards. Patients in the quiet wards do not like the doors to be thus arranged, as it takes from the privacy of their rooms; and the attendants' rooms ought certainly to have doors opening inwards, and the means of securing themselves from intrusion. A very simple precaution against the fastening of the door of the room by a patient in the inside is that of fixing the bedstead to the floor, which is easily done; and it is to be remembered that a door which opens outward may be burst open by a violent patient from within. All the doors in the wards assigned to violent patients should be of oak; and if they open outward, a few of the doors should have two locks, so placed as to prevent the yielding either of the upper or the lower part of the door to any force which the patient can apply. The ordinary cast-iron bedstead, when fitted up with a strong canvas bottom, hung on side rods, which readily draw out, so as to allow the removal of the canvas when required, is well adapted to many cases, even among the refractory and dirty; or, if desired, the crib bedstead, with the canvas stretcher, will suit the worst cases. These beds, as improved by Mr. Harris, at the Hanwell Asylum, are six feet long and three feet broad; and perhaps two or three inches more in length and width would be a further improvement. Whatever kind of bed is used, its perfect cleanliness is of the first importance. The sheets should be frequently changed, even in the cleanest wards, and daily, if required, in others. Want of sleep is sometimes occasioned by the patient being covered with old, hard blankets or coverlets, which confine the exhalations of the skin; and softer blankets and coverlets will remove the evil. The beds, whether made of coir, or horse-hair, or cotton-waste, or any other material, should not be allowed to become hard and knotty, but be frequently taken to pieces, washed, exposed to the air, and dried carefully. The patients who destroy blankets or bedding should be supplied with soft, warm blankets, properly protected, either by being quilted to ticking, or sewed up in a complete ticking-case.

In all asylums the proportion of single bedrooms appears to me to be too small; and I always recommend architects to have such rooms for at least two thirds of the number of patients to be received into any proposed asylum. A few dormitories, containing not more than four or five beds in each, are useful in an asylum. The timid and the melancholy are best placed in such rooms for the night, and those disposed to suicide are safer with others than alone. But in favour of large dormitories, I do not know one good reason that can be advanced. Those who sleep in them are generally discontented. The air of such large sleeping-rooms becomes indescribably oppressive when the patients have been two hours in bed; and it never becomes quite fresh and pure, although all the windows and doors are open, in the longest and finest day. One

One patient, accidentally noisy, disturbs the repose of fourteen or fifteen; and out of that number there is often some one noisy. One man suddenly irritated, or any one patient suddenly starting out of a dream, may rush on his nearest neighbour and injure him severely. Such accidents are very incidental to dormitories; and in those houses in which they are said to produce no inconvenience, I suspect that all who are likely to be troublesome are fastened to their beds. The violent patients must of course be in single rooms, and if dirty patients are herded together at night, a dormitory becomes perfectly disgusting: and as for the clean, and orderly, and tranquil, and convalescent patients, no complaint is so constantly on their lips as that which arises from their not having a single room, and, consequently, not having a single moment to themselves, or any place where they can be quiet, or, in their frequently uttered words, where they can even say their prayers without interruption. I would therefore have at least two thirds of the bedrooms single rooms, very few and small dormitories, and no large dormitories for any class of patients.

In the Derby plan the proportion of single bedrooms was rather less than two thirds; but the Commissioners condemned even this proportion as unnecessary. With great deference to the Commissioners, I consider this to be a serious mistake.

CHAPTER II.

Arrangement of Galleries and Sleeping-rooms.—Inspection-plates.—Doors and Windows.—Warming and Ventilation.—Lighting at Night.—Cleanliness.—Sources of Offensive Smells.—Dormitories, Water-closets, Sinks, &c. &c., their most convenient Arrangement.—Store-rooms.— Washing-rooms. — Baths. — Modifications required in Asylums for Patients of various Classes.

THE door of every bedroom at Hanwell is fitted up with what is called an inspection-plate, placed at so convenient a height that it may be looked through, if necessary, as the attendant passes along the galleries.   The plate is made of iron, and towards the gallery merely presents a flat surface and a small circular opening, over which there is a cover, which moves without noise, and may be fastened when desirable; the inside of the plate is broad and concave towards the patient's room, all parts of which thus become visible by looking through the opening from the outside.   These plates are convenient in every part of the asylum, but only absolutely necessary for rooms in which refractory patients are occasionally secluded in the daytime.   This little contrivance is connected with a very essential particular in the treatment of violent patients, being a means of ascertaining, from time to time, the state of any patient who is placed in temporary seclusion.   When the use of restraints was first forbidden, the safety of the attendants, and of the patients themselves, required that those in charge of the wards should have authority to place violent or unruly patients in their bedrooms for a time, locking the door.   By occasionally looking through the inspection-plate, the attendant is enabled to ascertain the effect of the seclusion; and the medical officers, to whom every seclusion is, or ought to be, immediately reported, are enabled to judge of the propriety of continuing or putting an end to it. We expect, when going through any gallery, to be informed what patients are in seclusion; and as the state of the patient can be immediately ascertained, a check is exercised over the abuse of an important remedial measure. The inspection-plate should be so made that the lid can be moved without the slightest noise; and a very little movement of it is sufficient. Some patients are peculiarly sensitive concerning being watched, and contrive to hang up clothes so as to obstruct inspection. This is chiefly the case with patients whom it is not necessary to look so closely after when left to themselves; but in the refractory wards the practice must not be permitted, or in the case of patients disposed to suicide. The inspection-plate at Hanwell is simple and efficient: the insertion of glass or wire in the opening, as sometimes recommended, would be attended with inconvenience; but as some patients are disposed to injure the eyes of the attendants when applied to the opening, a little caution is required, which is easily practised. In some foreign asylums, the patient's room is inspected through a window above the door; and for this the attendant requires a ladder; and the ladder has to be brought from the end of the gallery; so that the inspection cannot be expected to be very efficient. In other asylums, secret openings in the walls or roof have been proposed; but this, like most departures from simplicity of arrangement in an asylum, would seem to be a mere perversion of ingenuity. The active curiosity and sharpened senses of most of the patients would immediately discover these supposed secret openings; and they would be more likely to be offended by them than by a more avowed watchfulness, and would even triumph over the defeated contrivance. I have sometimes derived useful suggestions from intelligent patients, in the intervals between their paroxysms, respecting the management of others, or even of themselves, when refractory; and in most of such cases, all attempts at concealment or deception have been shown by their

observations to be eminently useless.   However troublesome
such patients may occasionally be, they know and appreciate
everything that is done, whether they are well or ill, and any
deceptions practised upon them are usually worse than
futile.

Another useful application of the inspection-plate is found
in its enabling us to ascertain the state of the sick and feeble,
or of the restless, whom it may have been desirable to leave
for a time undisturbed.   Patients in a very helpless state, or
patients who have just had violent epileptic attacks, are often
most securely placed in rooms in which there is a very low
bedstead, and no other furniture, or in rooms of which the
whole floor is covered with bedding.   Our padded rooms are
much more frequently required for such patients than for
violent patients, or for those disposed to strike their heads
against the wall.   Some of our paralytic patients, when reduced to a state of extreme helplessness, are placed in such
rooms, and several of our epileptics; but when restraints were
employed, such patients were fastened to common bedsteads,
often in loose straw, and became violent from excess of physical misery.   Restraint was the grand substitute for inspection,
superintendence, cleanliness, and every kind attention.   It was
not until restraints had been for some time abolished that I
ever found the inspection-plates properly attended to.   Troublesome patients were securely fastened down, and nobody
seemed to care what condition they were in.

It is desirable to have window-shutters to most or all of the
bedrooms.   They are indispensable in the bedrooms of refractory
wards, and should be made to shut easily, and to fasten with a
small spring-lock, or in some way which occasions no delay, and
so as not to be unfastened by the patients.   Sufficient light
should be admitted through perforations in the shutter to make
the inspection of a patient secluded in the daytime practicable.   Seclusion in total darkness is seldom, perhaps never, necessary; and it would often be a dreadful punishment, either
much aggravating the patient's agitation, or exciting frightful

thoughts. In visiting patients in private houses, I generally find the rooms made totally dark, but filled with anxious relatives, attendants, and half the servants of the house. All these things are unfriendly to the patient's tranquillity, and produce suspicion, fear, and increased violence. The locks of the bed-room doors should not be spring-locks, but simple locks, of a strong construction. There is great danger of injuring a patient who tries to come out of his room against the will of the attendant if the door fastens with a spring-lock; and the doors would, of course, be locked whenever closed, which would be highly inconvenient both to patients and attendants. The doors of the galleries should have spring-locks, without which they will seldom be locked at all. All the locks in the house should be so made, and so kept in order, as to open and close with the least possible noise. The jingling of keys, the clang of the locks, and the violent opening or shutting of the doors of bedrooms and galleries, are generally considered of no consequence by the attendants; but they produce the most uncomfortable feelings in the patients. The gallery doors should have large handles, enabling those who pass through to shut the door quietly. The state of a whole ward may immediately be altered by persons hastily and noisily passing through. There is, however, no point so little attended to by the generality of attendants, servants, workpeople, officers, and even by the official visitors of all asylums. The physician's caution is generally despised, and his example disregarded. Doors are thrown suddenly open; attendants are loudly or fiercely called for; unexplained intimations are given of something being wrong somewhere; the ward is hastily passed through; the hindering patients are put aside; the door is violently shut; the next ward and the next are similarly invaded; and the whole of the inmates, attendants as well as patients, are left in a state of agitation, or even of alarm. I have often, in former times, discerned the impression of these impetuous visits so distinctly left as to make me inquire into its cause; and have had deep reason to lament that it should be so much forgotten that the

manner, the voice, the words, the very step of those who pass
through a house full of insane people ought to be calm and
tranquillizing.   Those most conversant with the insane will
the most readily acquit me of exaggerating the importance of
these matters.   Being desirous, whenever I suggest arrangements which appear at first sight to be but remotely connected
with medical treatment, to append the reason to the suggestion,
my remarks on all points of building and construction become
unavoidably mingled with some details of treatment; for the
only standard I acknowledge in all the arrangements, is that
of their bearing on the patients.   There is no other test of
their goodness or badness.

No part of the subject of the construction of asylums is
more difficult to give a satisfactory opinion upon than that
which relates to the proper method of warming and ventilating
such buildings. Different plans are in use in different asylums,
and yet ventilation is generally found to be imperfect, and the
temperature of different parts of the building in winter very
unequal, varying in different wards as much, sometimes, as
twenty degrees of Fahrenheit.   If story is piled upon story,
and basement wards and dormitories are excavated, I believe
no system of ventilation will prevent the air of the asylum
from being generally unwholesome, and often highly offensive.
From subterranean dormitories insidious streams of corrupted
air are for ever rising, pervading every room above ground,
ascending every staircase, and infecting every corner. Visitors
go round such buildings in the middle of the day, and do not
perceive this, although in certain states of the weather it is
very perceptible ; but those who live in asylums, and who have
to return to them after breathing the fresh air of the evening,
or who visit the wards, and occasionally enter the bedrooms at
night, or who even pass the head of staircases leading to basement dormitories, in which the patients have been sleeping
two or three hours, know too well that the air becomes so im-
pure as sometimes to occasion immediate sickness;   and
although the governing bodies may persist in accumulating

beds wherever they can be placed, so close to each other as almost to touch, and subservient officers will permit these unsalutary practices, nothing is more certain than that all this is done at the expense of the general health of the whole establishment. In such asylums some of the attendants are always sick; febrile attacks, attended with great debility, are very common among them; what is called influenza becomes, as it were, domiciled and perpetual among them; and no one living under the roof of the asylum has the appearance of being in perfectly good health. Impaired health induces impaired spirits, and the efficiency of the attendants, and even of the officers, becomes manifestly diminished. They are too soon fatigued, and too easily dispirited; they are less comfortable, and less forbearing; and the final result of all these faults, and their consequences, is, that the patients suffer.

At Hanwell the ventilation is merely effected by the ordinary doors and windows, aided in some parts of the building by openings in the walls, or openings communicating with the roof. These openings, and some additional doors and windows in the basement story, have much improved the general ventilation of the building within the last few years, and it is seldom now that the heavy and peculiar atmosphere which used to pervade the wards is perceptible. The circular portions of the building, and the large dormitories in the basement, present the greatest difficulties in respect to efficient ventilation. Nearly the whole of the asylum is warmed by means of steam admitted into iron pipes, placed, in the older wards, about seven feet from the floor of the galleries, and in the newer parts, beneath the floor, and in some of the sleeping-rooms a little above the floor, inclosed in perforated wooden cases.

The chief objection to warming an asylum by steam is, that the warmth thus produced is very unequal in different parts of the building; oppressive in the wards nearest the boilers, and not sufficient in wards more remote; and that it also varies at different heights of the building. Generally speaking, the newest portions of the asylum, in which the steam-pipes are

beneath the floor, are the most comfortable in cold weather,
and the temperature appears to be more equally kept up in
them. The general coldness of the bedrooms is a great evil;
they never attain the warmth of the galleries, except when
steam-pipes are introduced into them. At night, except in
very severe weather, the steam is turned off, and the coldness
of some of the wards then, and in the morning when the patients are expected to get up, is extreme. It is difficult to
keep up the proper heat all night for the production of steam;
and this particular inconvenience may be avoided, by adopting
the plan of warming an asylum by means of hot-water pipes,
in which the water will circulate if its temperature is kept at
120° Fahr.   But this mode of warming is only applicable to
small buildings, and a general preference seems now given to
providing for the general warmth of a building by the admission, to all parts of the building, of air warmed by passing
over pipes containing hot water, provision being also made for
the passing out of foul air, either through simple openings in
the galleries and rooms, or through shafts containing fires, so
as to draw or pump out the used or foul air, and all the steam
and effluvia from the kitchen and other offices. This plan of
"air-drainage" is adopted in the plan for the Derby asylum;
and it is stated by Mr. Duesbury, that the areas of the flues,
and the rate of motion of the withdrawn and supplied air, will
be such as to secure a change of air of from sixty to one hundred feet per minute for each individual, the supply depending
on the variations of the general temperature.   The model
prison at Pentonville, the prison at Derby, and other buildings,
are already warmed and ventilated in this manner, which
seems peculiarly adapted to such buildings, as the prisoners
pass the greater part of the day, as well as the night, in their
cells.   It is possible that the complete ventilation of a well-
constructed and not over-crowded asylum may be effected
with a less elaborate apparatus, or, at least, without the
shafts.

But whatever mode of ventilating and warming an asylum

is adopted, it should be compatible with having the fresh air admitted unwarmed, and by open windows, in all temperate weather, and with having open fireplaces in every day-room, or, if there are no day-rooms, in every gallery, and in many of the work-rooms. Our windows at Hanwell do not admit air enough in the summer time; and advantage is gained in some asylums, as at Stafford, from having the glass of a part of the gallery or bedroom window set in wooden frames, corresponding in size and situation to iron frames placed exterior to them, so that the whole wooden frame can be opened without leaving the danger of an open window, and yet closed without any appearance of iron bars. When the wards are warmed by artificial means, there is too frequent a tendency to economize such means, by excluding the fresh air, and thus substituting warm, foul, and expired air, for fresh air warmed. This is one of the many faults which a specious economy too readily covers.

All my observation of the habits and condition of the insane at Hanwell has led me to be especially of opinion that whatever mode of warming is adopted, there is both utility and comfort in having fireplaces accessible to all patients, properly protected by a light iron guard, fastened with a small spring-lock. The inequality of temperature in different wards, and on different days, is a source of complaint all the winter; and in many autumnal days, as well as in the early spring, when the steam-warming or hot-air warming is discontinued, because it is no longer winter, or is not commenced because the winter has not yet come, the patients suffer excessively; and the feeble, elderly, paralytic, and epileptic are occasionally brought into a state of danger, only averted by removing them to a ward in which there is a comfortable fire. It is impossible to witness a party of lunatics sitting round a cheerful fire in winter, without wishing to see a fireplace in every ward. There is no comfort more missed by the poorest lunatic than that of an open fire, and many incidental conveniences are secured where this comfort is enjoyed. The visiting magistrates of Hanwell have lately authorized the introduction of fireplaces into most of the day-rooms, to the evident satisfaction of the patients. It would appear that the mere keeping of the general temperature of the galleries at 60° is not sufficient for comfort, and that much gratification arises from greater warmth being applied to the surface than is absolutely necessary for health. Our patients try to obtain this, even in the wards most efficiently warmed by steam, by lying down close to the gratings which admit the warmth; only imitating in this respect the general pleasure enjoyed by sane persons when they gather round a fireplace, although in warm apartments. The point becomes of more importance in relation to persons shut up in one place, and for whom the mere sight of a fire helps to break a daily monotony with difficulty imagined by those who are at liberty to go every day where they please.

I have mentioned fire-guards, although I know that they are disused in some asylums. I do not recommend their disuse in public asylums. Some patients are mischievous, and play with the fire dangerously; many are imbecile, and apprehend no danger from touching it; many are feeble, and may fall or be pushed into the fire; and some, debarred from other modes of self-destruction, may wilfully try to destroy themselves by burning. The guard should inclose the whole fireplace, but there should be a large opening in front, of which the lock should close of itself when the open part, or gate, is shut. If it requires to be locked by an attendant, this duty will often be forgotten. In the older asylums I have seen iron handcuffs hanging to the fire-guards, and to these, poor shivering wretches, half clothed and half starved, were fastened, if they came near the fire at all; being thus deprived of much of the comfort of being near the fire, and in some cases exposed to the danger of being half roasted. I even now occasionally see fire-guards in houses for the reception of insane gentlemen and ladies, of a form so clumsy, and so dismal, as to present a strong contrast to the light guards found efficient in asylums for the poor; and I observe that they are secured by a common padlock, which is objectionable both as regards appearance and convenience.

The manner in which the admission of light and air by the windows is made compatible with perfect security is illustrated in all asylums of recent construction. It is only in the older ones that windows are seen placed so high that no one can look out of them ; windows of small and scarcely transparent panes of glass, set in thick and heavy frames of wood, and guarded on the outside by massive bars of iron, precautions which may have been necessary in asylums where violence and neglect reigned uncontrolled, but which are utterly superfluous under existing modes of treatment. A very thick window-glass has recently been adopted in the bedrooms of some asylums, admitting a modified light, but which cannot be seen through : no invention can be more abominable. Our windows in the galleries and day-rooms at Hanwell are wide and cheerful, allowing the patients to look out as they sit at work. The panes are of good size, varying in different parts of the building from 10 inches by 6, to 8 inches by $5\frac{1}{2}$; and they are set in a light frame of cast iron, which is painted white. Towards the upper part of each window there is a circular portion with two sets of frames, one turning on the other, so as to leave open spaces, the glass being set in alternate spaces in each of the circles. In parts of the building in which there are small square windows, as in the rooms in the third story, the frame containing the upper row of panes turns on a swivel, so as to be partially opened ; but this kind of window is far from secure without the protection of wire-guards. Even the ordinary large windows, with a complete circle of panes capable of being opened, are not quite safe in bedrooms, unless there are shutters or wire-guards. The windows of the galleries of our refractory wards, and of some others, are guarded ; the rest without guards ; and on the male side, the experiment of having no window-guards in the day-rooms of two out of four of the refractory wards has been tried, without inconvenient results. In the Surrey Asylum I believe none of the windows are guarded; but if light honeycomb wire-guards are placed interiorly to the windows, so as to permit plants and birds to be put between the windows and the guards, the guards being painted white, and having a green frame, nothing unpleasant is offered to the eye. For the mere protection of the windows the guards should be about a foot from the glass. When restraints were first discontinued at Hanwell, the destruction of windows was said to be ruinous. I believe it was often most negligently permitted by attendants partial to the old means of securing the patients: now it has become quite trifling, having diminished with the decrease of all other kinds of violence and irregularity.

Window-frames of cast iron may be broken by a sharp and heavy blow with any hard instrument; and we had, some years ago, a patient who was very expert in doing this, and making his escape from the asylum; but such accidents can only happen where the attendants are negligent, and perhaps they are only likely to happen where patients are made unhappy by restraints. The patient alluded to was once or twice brought back to us. The period of emancipation from muffs and strait-waistcoats arrived in his time: he sometimes tried to provoke us to make him an exception, and to put restraints on him again; but he was treated differently, began to mend, got well, and was discharged cured. Since restraints were discontinued, I remember no instance of escape being effected by breaking the window-frames.

When these and worse accidents occurred at Hanwell, there was not an efficient window-shutter in the house. All kind of security had rested on fastening the arms and legs and bodies of refractory patients to bedsteads or to heavy chairs; and there was an interval between the removal of these fastenings and the supply of required shutters and other means, which interval was signalized by untoward occurrences, now seldom heard of in the asylum, and when occurring, attributable to some negligence of the same kind. Dr. Jacobi thinks that iron window-frames are attended with many other inconveniences, and seems much to prefer the old iron bars ; but his objections do not seem to be well founded. We do not find, at Hanwell, that the expansion or contraction of the iron ever breaks the panes, nor that they admit the air inconveniently, nor the rain generally ; nor do they darken the rooms, or open of necessity in a dangerous manner; nor do they stain and streak the glass in wet weather. The chief inconvenience, that of rendering it difficult to admit sufficient air through them in hot weather, has been already spoken of. The insertion of one pane of zinc in some of the windows, perforated for the admission of air, and making openings over the fireplaces, with a valve, permitting air to pass out of the ward also, as practised in some of the habitations of the poor in London, might perhaps remedy this fault.

The best method of lighting the galleries and day-rooms, as well as the chapel and larger apartments, in the winter evenings, is by coal-gas. If well prepared, it is the least offensive, and the cheapest kind of light. There should be several lights in each gallery and day-room, so placed as to enable the patients easily to read, write, work, or amuse themselves with cards, draughts, dominoes, &c. ; and one moderate light should be maintained in each gallery all night. There is a refinement of economy practised in some private asylums which grievously interferes with the comfort of educated patients, and which consists of allowing a long interval to elapse between the departure of daylight and the introduction of lamps and candles. A great amount of suffering is entailed on the patients by this ingenious neglect. This is generally allied with an equal anxiety to save in the article of fuel; and servants are permitted to forget to mend the fires with entire impunity. The same principle creeps sometimes into public asylums ; and to save the expenditure of a few shillings in a week, the patients are allowed to grope their way about the wards, and find their way to bed as they can, when the days are shortening, and when the patients are also cold and comfortless and irritable, in consequence of passing many hours in too low a temperature.

In whatever manner light and air are admitted into the wards, and warmth is diffused over the asylum, perfect cleanliness is indispensable. Nothing offensive to sight or smell should be permitted in any part of the asylum. Warmth must not be obtained by excluding the air, nor light by means corrupting the atmosphere. No excuse should be admitted for a bad smell in any room or corner. If perfect cleanliness cannot remove it from any one part of the building, there must be something wrong in the drainage or ventilation of that part, which ought to be rectified at any cost. But instances of this kind are few in comparison with the origin of such bad smells in neglect. Attendants who have not been well instructed in their duty, or who are not well affected to the non-restraint system, will stoutly maintain that this or that bed-room cannot be freed from a bad smell, do what they will; but such is scarcely ever the case, and for a proof that it is not the case, I would refer every visitor to Hanwell to the male ward No. 1. It is a ward in which every inconvenience has to be contended with; it is in the basement story; it has small windows; it has bed-rooms on both sides of the gallery, from one end to the other; it is the longest ward in the asylum, and it contains fifty patients, all of whom are imbecile or idiotic, many paralysed or helpless, and three fourths what are called dirty patients, requiring all the care of children. Four male attendants keep this ward so scrupulously clean that there is scarcely ever the least smell in any part of the gallery, or in any bedroom. The admirable cleanliness and general state of this particular ward are favoured by each patient having a single sleeping-room. If they slept in large dormitories, the air of the ward, and of all the wards above it, would become noxious to health. Dormitories in which only four or five dirty patients sleep are seldom free, even after being empty for many hours, from an odour offensive to a person who has a delicate sense of smell.

The provisions necessary for cleanliness are humble things to dwell upon, but they are the auxiliaries of health, and deserve the most vigilant attention of the physician, who ought to remember, when he detects a bad smell in passing any door in a gallery or passage, that some of the inmates of the asylum are exposed to that offensive air all the day long, and all the night, and that some of them never go out beyond the boundaries of the asylum grounds, so as to recruit, by change of air and scene, their constitutional power of resisting the influence of local malaria. And whoever pays much attention to the habits of human beings, must know how much the irritability of the mind is increased by habitual ill health, in whatever way produced; and it is with this irritability, on a large scale, that we have to deal, and which it is our business to remedy or prevent in asylums for the insane. It well illustrates the importance of everything in an asylum being regulated by the physician, when we find that even this point of cleanliness, so essential to health of body and mind, cannot be secured without well-chosen attendants. Their selection is allowed to rest at Hanwell, and in a few other asylums, with those who either do not understand or do not appreciate the comprehensive nature of the duties required by attendants, and the physician is compelled to work with inefficient instruments, and liable, any day in the week, and every week in the year, to find a great number of his patients deprived of the attentions of an efficient attendant, and placed at the command of those in whom it is impossible for him to place any confidence. But the subject of the selection, government, and duties of the ward-attendants will be subsequently treated of, with the fulness which its importance demands; and as I consider that I am addressing the public on subjects of more than ephemeral interest, I shall not abstain from condemning what is wrong, merely because it happens to be practised in the asylum to which I am myself the physician, and which I would fain see a model for general imitation.

The sources of bad smells in an asylum are chiefly the large dormitories already alluded to; the water-closets, sinks, and urinals, and also the neglected persons, and clothing or bedding of the patients. Until lately, the sinks in most asylums

were at once sinks, and watering-places, and washing-places.
The sinks should be used as sinks alone, and the door leading
to them should be locked by the attendants. There should be
in every ward a lavatory or washing-room, containing half-a-
dozen enamelled-iron washing basins, sunk in a leaden table,
and each basin supplied with a watercock, and having a
movable plug. There should also be one or two large round
towels in each room. Among the late additions to the wards
at Hanwell, none has been more productive of comfort to the
patients than this, and the washing-rooms are the perfection
of neatness. These rooms are open to the patients of quiet
wards at all hours of the day ; and the means of having a clean
face and hands, and the refreshment of washing when fatigued,
or after various occupations, is very much enjoyed. An additional means of personal cleanliness is also afforded by each
patient having a warm bath once a week. Where these regulations prevail, the skin of insane patients loses its most re-
pulsive and unwholesome aspect ; general health is promoted,
and with health, comfort, and cheerfulness ; and the peculiar
odour of the insane, so often described, does not permeate
every ward, and is, indeed, seldom perceived. There are private asylums, on the old plan, which I could recognize as such,
if taken blindfolded into them ; and where this terrible and
peculiar smell tells the visitor, as plainly as any impression on
the sense can tell, that the rooms are not thoroughly clean,
that the bed and body linen are not sufficiently often changed,
and that washing and bathing are very little attended to.

Every ward of an asylum should have one room in it appropriated to keeping the clothing and linen required for the
immediate use of the ward ; and although certain general rules
for the supply of clean linen must be observed, these rules
must have many exceptions in favour of the patients. In or
near every ward there should be a bath-room, containing one
or two baths, raised above the floor, and of moderate depth.
When many patients are required to take baths at the same
time, the baths may even be shallow ; their depth at Siegburg

is one foot five inches, their length five and a half feet, and their width two feet. The best material for the bath is stone, painted, and the edges rounded. There should be a matting, or rug, or carpet at the side of the bath when it is used. It is convenient to have the head of the bath towards a wall, and the two sides and the foot of the bath free, so that, when required, the attendants can stand round the patient. The best method of supplying the water is by a single opening at the bottom of the bath, admitting hot and cold water at the same time. The handles to turn the water off or on should be out of the patient's reach. To avoid the difficulty and pain attending the removal of feeble and bedridden patients to the bath-room, we had some slipper-baths at Hanwell placed on wheels, but they were not often employed. In the hospital of St. Louis, at Turin, (for incurable maladies,) there is a door behind each bed, and each bed is on wheels, so as to be moved, if required, to the bath-room. Shower-baths of moderate force are so often useful, that I should always prefer having an apparatus for one fixed over each bath. To be effective, they should be supplied from a large cistern, or reservoir. The ordinary shower-baths, only containing from seven to ten gallons of water, and which are filled slowly and with difficulty, are very troublesome, and are more fitted for refreshment or gentle excitement, than for subduing violent symptoms. As it is extremely difficult to keep a refractory patient under the shower, it is useful to have a few shower-baths made of a square shape, and inclosed; the upper half of the door being made of wirework, and the whole of the top of the bath perforated. Some of our bath-rooms at Hanwell are fitted up with a leaden pipe, to which a hose-pipe can be affixed, for the purpose of administering the douche-bath; but I have long ceased to employ this form of bath, which occasions much more distress to the patient than the shower-bath, without any corresponding advantage.

No care can be too great to keep the water-closets within the building, and the outside privies, and the urinals, free from offensive accumulations and bad smells. All urinals are invariably offensive unless there is a small stream of water continually running over their surface. Privies out of doors are required in courts where very maniacal patients, or imbecile patients, take exercise; but in the airing-courts for the more comfortable patients they are superfluous. If there is a deep fall, there should be the security of a grating, to prevent the patients from leaping down; and if there is very little depth under the seat, the accumulation becomes highly inconvenient. All privies become sources of trouble and annoyance, unless made on the principle of a water-closet, or, at least, unless a powerful stream of water can be commanded, to carry away all accumulations. An abundant, never-failing supply of water is the great requisite for cleanliness, and to secure it no expense should be spared. It creates a benefit for ever. The asylum at Siegburg is for 200 patients, and it is computed by Dr. Jacobi that 4014 gallons of water are required daily. For the use of the Hanwell asylum, containing 1000 patients, we require 40,000 gallons of water per diem, or about double the proportion allowed at Siegburg; and at the cost of 1000*l.* a deep well has been formed, which supplies 100 gallons per minute at the surface, and about 20 gallons per minute 26 feet above the surface. When there is this abundant supply of water, I prefer, to all others, the plan of water-closet by which a current of water is carried through it whenever the door is opened and shut. The supply then depends on no one's attention, and no one's caprice, but there may possibly be some waste of water. When the current of water depends on the pressing down of the seat, and the subsequent removal of the pressure, various accumulations of an offensive kind may occur, from things poured into the closet without any pressure of the seat being made. The dependence of the current of water on the pulling of a string, or lifting up and depressing a handle by an attendant, is sure to lead to neglect. Even in private houses, it is well known that without constant care the water-closets infect the whole house.

All arrangements in an asylum for the insane, I would once more observe, and particularly those relative to doors, windows, and window-shutters, fire-guards, ventilators, baths, and water-closets, should be as simple and uncomplicated as possible. If much trouble is occasioned by opening and closing the window-shutters, or fire-guards, or ventilators, the trouble will be as often as possible avoided. Even when a fire-guard shuts with a spring-lock, the attendants will not take the trouble to close it, because in an hour or two they may have to employ a key to open it. Officers of asylums are sometimes prone to overload the attendants with minute duties, and the consequence is a neglect of some that are more important.

The observations included in the present chapter have reference principally to County Asylums for Pauper Lunatics. In asylums for the classes above them, many modifications of the architect's plan are necessary. Several private sitting-rooms are required; and these may be on the ground-floor, and open into gardens, or into a gallery or corridor; the bedrooms must almost all be single rooms, opening into a gallery above-stairs. Various other arrangements become obviously requisite, according to the rank of the patients, and their habits of living, and the extent of accommodation required by them. But the general principles of arrangement must be the same : there must be the same general attention to the health of the intended inmates; and there must be apartments for the refractory, the noisy, and the dirty, although the furniture may be of different materials from those used in a pauper asylum. Where such arrangements are not adopted, restraint is the general substitute for them; and the richer patient is more unfavorably situated than the poorer lunatic, and is, indeed, not unfrequently treated with excessive cruelty.

Many of Dr. Jacobi's remarks on the construction of asylums contemplate providing in the same asylum for patients of differect ranks, or of all ranks. But asylums built for the re-

ception of both rich and poor patients can never be free from
many objections; and the uncomfortable suspicion is inseparable from them—that the humbler patients have the refuse
of the provisions, and the most indifferent attendance. If
such a mixture of classes in one asylum should be unavoidable,
the establishments for the different classes ought to be vir-
tually distinct, although in immediate contiguity, as in the
new asylum near Glasgow.

The buildings and arrangements in the greater number of
private asylums continue to be very defective. Gloom and
confinement seem to be inseparable from an ordinary private
dwelling when made into an asylum; and the cheerless aspect,
the faded furniture, the want of fresh air, and of proper
warmth and light, and of free egress to the courts or gardens,
and even, too often, of proper attention to cleanliness, are op-
pressively conspicuous. Some assimilation in these respects,
and in others, to the plan and arrangements of public asylums,—
due attention being given to the requirements of patients who
have been accustomed to enjoy every kind of comfort, and to
the feelings of their friends on these points,—would greatly
improve many of them.

CHAPTER III.

Situation of Wards for the Elderly and Feeble.—Infirmaries.—Former Abuses of Restraints in Wards for the Sick.—Present Arrangements.— Airing Courts and Grounds.—Classification out of doors.—Recreations without and within doors.—Evening Entertainments.—Clothing of the Insane.

In the arrangement of an asylum, peculiar provision should be included for the elderly and feeble, of which the number is generally increasing in asylums in which the incurable patients remain for life. Quiet, airy wards, on the ground-floor, should be allotted to these weak and old people, with doors opening into grassy airing-courts. Above these wards, the infirmaries for the sick, the paralytic, and others whose strength is rapidly declining, may conveniently be placed. Perhaps the most advantageous situation for all these wards for the old and weak and sick would be a small retreating wing at the extremity of the main line of the building, where the advancing wings also commence.

It is incredible to what an extent all provision of this kind seems to have been forgotten in asylums for the insane, until within the last few years. Even at Hanwell, the whole design of which was dictated by humanity, and arose out of the anxiety of benevolent persons to deliver pauper lunatics from the dens in which they were before confined, the sick were for a time placed in small close wards, in a third story, at the two extremities of the building; being the wards the most difficult of access, and from which the sick could scarcely get out of doors for air or exercise; placed, too, the most remotely from the chapel, the surgeries, and the kitchen, and over the refractory and dirty wards, with which they communicated

by an open staircase. No places could have been more
unfortunately selected for the sick, less convenient to the
medical officers and attendants, or more exposed to disturbance and to bad air. This was the simple result of an
habitual forgetfulness that the insane required some treatment
beyond mere confinement in galleries and bedrooms. As it
always happens that among patients recently affected, some
are sick and feeble, and likely to die, and are yet, at the same
time, occasionally violent, the infirmaries had gradually
become places in which restraint was more abused, and more
frequently and more repulsively employed, than in any other
parts of the asylum. The consequences were, that physical
suffering and mental disorder were alike aggravated, and the
severest methods of repression resorted to in wards where
attention to sickness ought to have been the principal duty of
the officers. Violence, noise, refusal of food, destruction of
bedding, tearing away of dressings, a disposition to suicide,
and all other irregularities, productive of daily agitation, now
past and even unknown, but never to be forgotten, were then
more frequently witnessed in the infirmaries than anywhere
else. I never enter those two wards, now assigned to a
different class of patients, without recollecting the miserable
struggles, the violence, and the wretched death-bed scenes,
characteristic of a time when restraints were so familiarly
employed, and so perseveringly kept on, as not even to be
removed until life was extinct. Those who now visit the
asylum, and who witness no such scenes, may be excused for
imagining that I am needlessly apprehensive of the use of
restraints being revived, and may talk, with apparent reason-
ableness, of the occasional and moderate employment of such
methods. Experience has taught me that their shocking
abuse, if once more witnessed, would subvert all such
reasonings. Their abuse, to an extent which now can scarcely
be described without a suspicion of exaggeration, and in an
asylum distinguished from its first opening by the comforts
and advantages it extended to the pauper lunatic, shows that

their use, to any extent, cannot be permitted without danger. Attendants trained in asylums where restraints are used, immediately apply them in private and recent cases, thus producing the worst consequences. Of this I meet with frequent and lamentable instances in private practice; where days, precious to the treatment of recent cases, are passed in all the misery and disadvantage of bonds, and dirt, and darkness, and unregarded fever, restlessness, and thirst.

It was in the female infirmary at Hanwell, exactly seven years ago, that I found, among other examples of the forgetfulness of what was due either to the sick or insane, a young woman lying in a crib, bound to the middle of it by a strap round the waist, to the sides of it by the hands, to the foot of it by the ankles, and to the head of it by the neck: she also had her hands in the hard leather terminations of canvas-sleeves; she could not turn, nor lie on her side, nor lift her hand to her face; and her appearance was miserable beyond the power of words to describe. How long she had been in this state it is not material to record. That she was almost always wet and dirty, it is scarcely necessary to say. But the principal point I wish to illustrate by mentioning this case is, that it was a feeble and sick woman who was thus treated. At that very time, her whole skin was covered with neglected scabies, and she was suffering all the torture of a large and deep-seated abscess of the breast. Let it be considered what must be the effect on the attendants of having customary recourse to the imposition of restraints, when such complicated suffering as this became comparatively disregarded by medical men, in consequence of the spectacle presented to them being, at each visit, not that of a sick person requiring aid, but of a dangerous lunatic cruelly fastened and bound. But this patient was neither dangerous to herself nor to others. The excuse alleged for this mode of treatment was, that she would eat the poultices employed, and which contained lead, and that she was very mischievous: that was all. However, she was liberated; no bad consequences ensued, and in a few

weeks I saw the poor creature at the chapel, and even heard
her play the organ, which she had been accustomed to do in
the church of a village in Middlesex before her admission.
This patient died very recently; having from the time of her
liberation from restraints scarcely ever given any trouble to
the attendants.   Perhaps if I had never seen such a case, I
should have been less earnest to adopt the system which I
knew had been tried at Lincoln, and slower to try to manage
the patients of this great asylum entirely without restraints.
Many a case was yet to be managed in which every ingenious
difficulty was created or encouraged to baffle this attempt;
many anxieties were to be endured, many misapprehensions
to be submitted to, and much suffered : but all is now passed ;
and I thank God, with deep and unfeigned humility, who has
permitted this great experiment to proceed, for full seven
years, without one accident calculated to discredit it ; and
with a general result on the asylum best known to those who
knew the asylum before ; and a general effect on all other
asylums in almost every region of the globe, which can never
be entirely lost.   Gratefully acknowledging the assistance
derived from the officers who supported me in this attempt,
and the visiting justices, who uniformly defended the great principle of it, I shall mention, with reluctance, any faults yet
existing in this noble institution, and not without a sanguine
hope of their eventual removal.

Our infirmaries now present a very different character, and
the patients have the benefit of many comforts,—kindness,
careful watching, tranquillity, religious consolation, and
friendly words ; and every soothing means conducive to relief
of bodily suffering, and to peace of mind.   No noise, no violence, no imprisonment, no bonds are there to be seen or
heard ; but in their place all that the sick and weak require,
furnished, literally without limitation, on the recommendation
of the medical officers.   Although the worst and most helpless cases are sometimes necessarily admitted there, with all
the increasing infirmities of declining power and life, both the

infirmaries are always scrupulously clean. Beds of various kinds are found there, adapted to the feeble, to those suffering from ulcerations of the back, and to the bedridden, and those who have sustained serious accidents. A chair and a small table by the side of each bed enable the attendants to leave water or other refreshing drinks within the patient's reach; and books, and pictures, and flowers, often show that friendly visitors have sate by the bedside, mindful of the alleviations to which even the insane are generally sensible. These visits I always encourage. There cannot be too many kind people about the insane in their hours of sickness and weakness; and I regard with abhorrence any attempts made to exclude such visitors, and even the kind members of the families of the officers, from the wards, on the plea of their having no official duties to perform.

I regret to have to mention that attempts of this kind have, within my own experience, been exclusively made by the matrons of asylums; more jealous, I fear, of their personal influence than anxious for the consolation of the patients.

Easy seats, sofas, and low safe arm-chairs, have also superseded benches and chairs of coercion in our infirmaries. The most careful provisions for warmth, a liberal daily diet, food and cordials, administered in the night, as well as by day, by attendants enjoined never to allow the infirmary patients to be left; and the means, for those able to walk, or requiring to be drawn about in wheeled chairs, of getting out of doors without great difficulty; all attest that the attention of the medical officers has taken a salutary direction, and that the cure and relief of the patients is the great principle observed in the infirmaries, and throughout the house.

Both with reference to health and recreation, as well as to employment, the airing-courts and grounds and gardens of an asylum are worthy of especial attention. A most gratifying improvement has taken place in these respects also, within the last few years, in many asylums. In the older institutions these had no place, or dismal yards and barren courts

3

were alone to be seen.   No external influence could have been
devised more powerful to depress the mind, and sink it into
inactivity, than monotonous gravel courts, surrounded by
walls from ten to fifteen feet high; without a tree; without a
shrub; without a blade of grass; without shade in the heat
of summer, or shelter from the rains of winter—the only
luxury being a bench fastened to the wall, with large iron
rings suspended over it, so that even in the open air restraint
might still be substituted for superintendence.   In these
respects, asylums were, until very lately, precisely like jails,
in one of which a man, who had been long imprisoned for an
act committed in a fit of insanity, used to say to me, when I
visited him,—" Sir, I have not seen a flower or a green leaf
these seven years !"—a painful observation to the ears of those
who can pass from such gloomy precincts to fields and
pleasant footpaths, never more to be trodden by the miserable.
Within equally melancholy boundaries might be seen, in most
asylums, but a few years ago, every form of gloom and eccentricity which the absence of all external objects of interest
could foster; and the patients walked up and down some
chosen path beneath the hopeless walls, until the very ground
was worn into hollows ; or, debarred from the full exercise of
the muscles of locomotion required by their excited brain
and nerves, expended all their energy in exertions of voice,
distressing to all within hearing.   Even at present, such
arrangements may yet be witnessed, and the consequent con-
centration of morbid excitement of a crowd of insane people,
which ought rather to be allowed relief by action and expansion in liberal space.

As a general rule in an asylum, every patient capable of
moving about should be out of doors at least an hour or two
every day, and the most active, who yet cannot be regularly
employed, should be out several hours.   Careless attendants
will avail themselves of the general indolence of the patients,
and neglect to take them out; and the officers of asylums
sometimes merely attach importance to making the patients

work, and disregard their taking other exercise : but nothing
has so great a tendency to increase the irritability of the
patients as keeping them within doors. , The value of opportunities of enjoying air and exercise has long been recognized
by the committee at Hanwell, and they have been so duly
impressed with the remedial advantages of airing-grounds, as
to have directed a series of alterations—the effecting of which
has occupied several years, and of which the object has been,
to make the airing-courts and the large fields in front of the
asylum more convenient and more cheerful. Nearly every
airing-court has been converted into a garden, and an abundant portion of ground assigned to the entire use of the most
tranquil and orderly patients. Shrubs and trees have been
planted, which promise shade and refreshment for years to
come ; summer-houses have been erected, and numerous seats
scattered about, where the female patients may rest, or the
male patients smoke their pipes in peace : and all who know
the Hanwell patients intimately can appreciate the positive
happiness thus conferred upon many of the tranquil and
incurable, whom modern views would consign to the comfortless yards of workhouses. In the fine days of the year,
hundreds of our patients are to be seen out of doors, enjoying a freedom most agreeable to contemplate, and seldom
abused. Even the lowering of the walls of the airing-courts
from ten feet in height to seven, has been appreciated by
some of the patients, who seldom go into the front fields, as
admitting a wider view of neighbouring trees, and a freer air.
In front of the asylum, the high embankment of the Great
Western Railway has indeed shut out from all the windows
of the asylum one of the most pleasing views in Middlesex ;
but some compensation is found for this in the frequent
passing of the railway-trains, by which no excitement is produced, and the patients are reminded that they are not quite
removed from the more varied and busy world, but only
sheltered from its cares. The general effect of all these
arrangements on the health of the patients of an asylum is

undoubted.   Those who are excited are induced to walk
about, and exercise gives them relief.   The reluctance of the
more numerous class of the indolent and apathetic to moving
out of the galleries or day-rooms is often overcome by an invi-
tation to walk in the field or the garden, and sometimes a certain number of the female patients walk into the orchards
with a nurse, and are found to be interested in the progress
of the fruit and vegetables.   Under proper regulation, this
indulgence ought frequently to be allowed.   The cultivation
of the gardens, and of the ground called the farm, as well as
of the extensive ornamental ground in front of the asylum,
is entirely effected by the labour of numerous male patients,
superintended by gardeners, or by steady workmen.   The
cheerfulness with which their work is performed, and the
satisfaction with which, at stated hours, they assemble for
their allowance of beer, sufficiently attest that calming and
remedial influences are thus exercised.   By occupying many
patients out of doors, the galleries and day-rooms become
comparatively empty during a great part of the day, and are
more perfectly ventilated, whilst those patients who are not
disposed to go out, or are too excited to be taken out with the
rest, enjoy comparative quietness in the wards.

The larger exercising-grounds of asylums should always
contain summer-houses, flower-borders, wide gravel walks
between rows of lime-trees, or other trees of quick growth,
not obstructing the proper inspection of the patients when
walking there.   A bowling-green, a cricket-ground, seats
under the trees, and the encouragement of ball-playing, or
hoop or battledore, or trap-ball, or ninepins, are all worth
remembering ; and buildings containing birds of various
kinds, and tame animals, will be found to interest many of
the patients.   A piece of shallow water, with ducks and other
aquatic fowl, would also give them pleasure.

To make the airing-courts agreeable to those patients who
are not employed, and who are less active, is not always easy.
The court should be so disposed in relation to the building

that the classification attempted within doors should be maintained out of doors also. Each ward should communicate
with an airing-court containing no other patients, and patients
of tranquil wards should not overlook the patients of refractory wards, or be overlooked by them, or even be within hearing of them. To effect this in an asylum of moderate extent,
and only two stories in height, is difficult; but in a larger
asylum, with more stories, it is impossible. The walks should
be wide, and made of fine well-rolled gravel, and there should
be shrubs, and flower-beds, and mounds, and sheltered seats.
It is part of the plan of the Derby Asylum to have in each
airing-court a paved arcade for exercise, and a pavilion with
seats at the end; the airing-courts are also to be surrounded
by a sunk wall, affording to the patients a view of the surrounding country. The airing-grounds at Lincoln have this
great advantage. Where higher walls are necessary they may
be covered with plants.

In the airing-courts for the more mischievous of the patients,
shrubs and trees are not so useful, and are sometimes inconvenient. Great care should be taken in the preparatory
drainage of airing-courts, otherwise the patients must be kept
within doors on many fine days, or parts of days, in winter,
in consequence of their disposition to dabble in the pools of
dirty water. I cannot approve of paving airing-courts, even
for the refractory, with flag-stones, and I believe that wood-
pavement, or caoutchouc, would be found very objectionable.
Nothing is so agreeable in all weathers as smooth gravel, care
being taken to remove all the larger stones, and to roll the
gravel diligently after rain. But in an asylum possessing
proper means of subdivision, the number of patients requiring
to be in airing-courts of mere gravel would be extremely
small, as, indeed, the number of really refractory patients
becomes under good regulations. Our four wards for refractory patients on each side of the house, and which contain
altogether about two hundred patients, seldom exhibit more
than ten or twelve on each side, who, either from their rest-

lessness or want of intelligence, are really turbulent at the same time; indeed, on the male side, out of four hundred patients, it is rare to find five turbulent at the same time; and at Lincoln, where the number of patients is much smaller, and the treatment consequently more individualized, I have been informed by Dr. Charlesworth, that the wards for the refractory are either occupied by very few patients, or are entirely empty. The wards called refractory in the Hanwell Asylum are on many days the most orderly wards in the house. They are generally the best attended to by the attendants.

In devising out-of-door recreation, it is necessary to avoid such as would endanger heedless patients, or be capable of being turned to mischievous purposes. Swings, see-saws, roundabouts, and various diversions popular at fairs, are on these accounts scarcely to be recommended. The large rock-ing-horses to be seen in all our airing-courts at Hanwell are free from all objection. Five or six patients can safely ride upon them at once, or one patient can be amused by them; the free exercise they afford relieves the excited, and the gentle motion which single patients, sitting in the seat at their ends, can enjoy, often soothes them to sleep. Means of amusement out of doors are useful to the attendants as well as to the patients; they contribute to relieve the irksomeness of their duties, and act as inducements to their taking the patients out as often as they can.

Within doors similar care should be extended to providing recreation for the patients during the winter days and even-ings. Each ward in which the patients are generally tranquil, should be provided with books, journals, magazines, illustrated papers, picture-albums, bagatelle, and draught-boards, domi-noes, cards, puzzles, soft balls, and even some descriptions of playthings; and the supply of these means of amusement should be carefully kept up. If music is encouraged among the patients, kind people will be found to furnish instruments which could not properly be bought for a county asylum.

There are three pianos at Hanwell, two of which were presented by friends of the institution known to myself. Flutes,
clarionets, and violins have occasionally been bought for patients who could play. Some of the attendants are tolerable
musicians, and a small band has been formed, which contributes much to the enjoyment of the winter-evening parties.
It is by no means uncommon, on approaching the wards appropriated to the more troublesome patients, on the male side
of the asylum, to hear a lively performance on the fiddle, and
to find patients dancing to it. Large musical boxes, or small
hand-organs might occasionally be taken into particular wards
with benefit. A few years ago it was the custom to have a
music evening once a week, which was looked forward to with
great pleasure by both the male and female patients ; but
these depended for their success on the zeal of resident officers
and their families, who have now left the asylum. The female
patients often have small parties for dancing, and there are
some entertainments on a larger scale, which have often been
described. For these there ought to be a large apartment in
every asylum, which might be otherwise useful also. In or-
dering these entertainments, the object should always be to
produce gratification to the patients, without hurtful excitement. This is admirably effected in the evening entertainments, and as much forgotten in the extremely objectionable
publicity of what are called fancy-fairs, which ostentatious
amusements, however well fitted to the idle and frivolous who
are at large, are quite inconsistent with the character of an
asylum for those suffering from mental disorder. In a well-
ordered asylum, the attendants should be encouraged to learn
singing and music, so that their means of amusing the patients
may be increased. This was attempted at Hanwell, but put a
stop to, as well as the schools, in accordance with views which
had not my approval, and, indeed, without any reference to
my opinion or wishes.

It is difficult for the physician to an asylum to make others
comprehend how important many influences, in themselves

apparently trifling, become, when the aggregate of their operation is continually applied to disordered minds. Vulgar
approbation is easily obtained by occasional display, although
the general character of an asylum may be that of a mere
workhouse or place of safety, in which nothing is habitually
done, beyond employing the patients, and keeping them quiet,
for their recovery. The faults of commission may be few, and
of omission many. The wards may be generally quiet. There
may be a solitude falsely called peace. Contrivance may secure this at all ordinary hours of public inspection, and especially on committee-days, and yet the hours of rising, and of
going to bed, and of meals, may be often signalized by irregularities and violence, and the patients may pass a very large
part of their time unoccupied, unamused; their hourly comforts little cared for—their recreations quite disregarded; so
that many of them become more and more listless, and even
at length incurable from neglect. No reflecting and experienced physician can walk through the wards of any large
asylum without seeing proofs of this; and for the effectual
counteraction of such an evil, and the calling forth of daily
and hourly resources yet unemployed, there seems to be required an energy and ingenuity on the part of superintendents, seconded by proper authority over a sufficient number
of officers and assistants, such as cannot yet be freely exercised
in any asylum. Much therefore remains to be done, which
cannot be done at present.

I must again observe that all the arrangements which I
have recommended, and all other arrangements for the health
and comfort of the insane, can only be effectual as a part of
one great and uniform system, of which humanity, and an
anxiety to cure or to relieve the patients, constitute the vital
principle. It is in vain to attempt to attach them to the old
system of restraints, and wholly impracticable to permit the
freedom of exercise, and the variety of diversion which have
been mentioned, without such a constant and well-ordered
superintendence as never yet existed, and never will exist in

an asylum where restraints are habitually trusted to. We expect, at Hanwell, as constant a care of the patients, and as vigilant an attention to their dress, their language, and their conduct, when taking exercise, as when in the wards. The attendants are required to be so placed as to maintain a continual observation of the whole of the ground, and of every patient, and no improper licence is ever permitted. This enables us to indulge many very lively, and some even rather excited patients, in various active amusements in the open air: others are attracted to come out by the variety thus presented to them; and some of the sick are carried out, or drawn out in the invalid chairs; so that some share of benefit is extended to all the patients. The excited or irritable become tranquillized, the melancholy and pensive have their thoughts for awhile diverted, and the imbecile are amused.

It is the same with the evening parties. The first sight of three hundred insane persons, assembled for an entertainment, and stimulated by a lighted and decorated apartment, and the presence of strangers, and the sound of music, and allowed to dance as freely, and even as fantastically, as each may choose, is one which an unfamiliar spectator can scarcely witness without feeling some immediate trepidation. But in an asylum where kindness is the rule, and where all the officers and all the attendants, and even the visitors, are known to entertain cordial feelings towards the patients, and where the patients are unaccustomed to any kind of violent treatment, or even to sharp or unkind reproof, it is found that a character of order prevails, which is not lost sight of amidst the excitement of the liveliest dancing and enjoyment. What appears to be an almost unrestrained activity is moderated by one timely, kind, and judicious word; and excitement which seems likely to transgress due bounds, is suspended in a moment by friendly conversation. When the hour of separation arrives, cheerful faces and grateful expressions show the general good effect of the indulgences accorded, on which, usually, sound sleep is found speedily to ensue. Such are the

3 §

general effects; and the especial effects on some of the patients are even more remarkable.

Instead of affecting to dictate to architects in relation to details better understood by themselves, I would wish to direct their attention, as well as that of the governing committees of asylums, to these, the real uses of airing-grounds and airing-courts, and rooms for entertainments; for when once the application is fully understood, the benefits required may doubtless be obtained in various ways, and the plans of future asylums may be improvements on the best now existing. These are among the advantages which it is proposed to give to the poor lunatic by county asylums; and they cannot be commanded in workhouses, or any small establishments instituted with a mere view to the saving of expense. The pauper lunatic is not merely to be secured; he is, if possible, to be restored to reason. To provide for the pauper lunatic is also not a mere duty; it is an enlarged charity; and the benevolence by which hospitals and dispensaries for the sick are supported, should by no means be withheld from asylums, which are the only hospitals for the sick and wounded in mind.

It is astonishing to find that one of the particulars of treatment in which the rich patient is sometimes more unfavorably situated than the poor, is that of having the opportunity of enjoying free and frequent exercise. The untrodden lawn, the dusty and desolate courts, the paved yards, the wretched sheds, the lonely outhouses, together with the closed doors and windows of a private asylum, often give to such places an external character which makes the visitor regard them with dread, and the passer-by speak of them in whispers. The idea of their entrance is connected with that of the fatal gate, which whoso entered left all hope behind. If a patient is visited in such a house, the unlocking of doors, and the threading of long passages, and ascent of gloomy stairs, with the close atmosphere of apartments filled with patients sitting by the walls, oppressed with indolence and monotony, are all features too familiar to those who knew such houses before later improvements penetrated into them. And it is only in a few of the best private asylums that we even now find cheerful sitting-rooms on the ground floor, opening on gardens, into which the patients may walk when they please; and the benefit of this improvement is yet too generally limited to the most rational of the patients, and not extended to the irritable and troublesome, who ought also to be able to go out of their sitting-rooms, although into gardens more secluded and secure. The extent of ground assigned to the patients, their subdivision during exercise, and, indeed, all the other arrangements in private asylums, vary so much in different establishments in these days of movement, that the remarks justly applicable to several which have adhered to the ancient ways, would be most unjust, as well as painful, to the proprietors of some, in which no sacrifice has been spared to secure for every patient all the advantages which a physician or a conscientious superintendent would wish them to enjoy. The excellence of the houses, the extent and variety of the grounds, the provision made for carriage and horse exercise, as well as for diversified walks, and for many kinds of recreation and amusement suitable to persons of education and of a certain rank, are such in a few of the private asylums, both of England and of France, as scarcely to leave anything to be desired; except, perhaps, the advantage yet to be added to the best existing modes of treatment, by means of well-educated auxiliaries, in addition to the ordinary attendants; persons capable of acting as guides, companions, and friends to those so much needing guidance, companionship, and friendly encouragement and care in every step of doubtful convalescence.

The clothing of the patients in an asylum of any description merits very careful attention, both as one of the means of preserving health, and as one of the things reacting on the mind. Among the most constant indications of insanity are to be observed negligence or peculiarity as to dress; and many patients seem to lose the power of regulating it according to the seasons, or the weather, or the customs of society. As regards the clothing of the pauper lunatic in a county asylum, it is especially desirable that it should be warm, both in the winter and in the changeable weather of the autumn and spring, and cool and unirritating in the summer. The vernal excitement so distinctly visible in the wards, seems to suggest particular attention to the clothing at the season when the temperature becomes rather suddenly elevated, after the severities of the winter and early spring. The irritability of some of the patients, and the coldness and increased feebleness of others, show the importance of warm winter clothing for patients suffering from various forms of nervous disturbance, which seem frequently to interfere with the function of animal heat. Without great attention to the clothing, both as regards its character and state, several paralytic patients would suffer severely, and even lose their lives. Many of the insane, also, are predisposed to pulmonary consumption, and a flannel waistcoat or drawers are indispensable to them, as well as to those who become depressed and inactive in severe weather. Warm worsted stockings, and cloth boots or shoes, kept in good repair, are very essential to some of them. The slovenly character given to most of the imbecile and maniacal patients by the falling down of their stockings over the ankles might be avoided, I imagine, by the structure of the upper part of the stocking being assimilated to that of children's half-stockings, which are easily kept up; or an elastic band at the top of the stocking might be convenient. Garters are generally lost or misapplied, and strings are inconvenient or useless. In these matters, the physician should be aided by female sub-officers, willing to learn, and ready to assist. Boots made of cloth are much worn at Hanwell, and seem very useful; if necessary, they are fastened on by a small lock, instead of a button. Stout linen is the material used both for men's shirts and women's under garments at Hanwell. Some of the female patients, unaccustomed to coarse apparel, complain of the skin being irritated by the linen, and calico is occasionally.

substituted for it. The men have clean shirts twice a week, and the attendants and officers should not permit them to be worn without buttons. A great number of the patients will keep themselves clean and neat if allowed to do so, and they should be in every respect assisted and encouraged in it. The best outer clothing for both the male and female patients in winter is woollen cloth. A gray broadcloth is worn at Hanwell by the men, and gray linsey gowns are worn by the women; but some of the women find a woollen gown oppressive, especially if they are employed; and cotton dresses, or linen check, of various patterns, or merino dresses, are provided for them. In the summer, the woollen gowns are certainly too warm, except for very weak and inactive patients. The number of female patients who go about bareheaded is always greatest where there is the most neglect. It is not natural to the woman to neglect the dress of her head, and if the faculty is impaired, care will often restore it. When convalescence is commencing, the patient generally becomes more cheerful if some assistance is given her as regards her dress for Sunday; and of this a neat, or even a pretty cap, is an important part. The men also, when recovering, often ask for newer clothing to go to chapel in. The attendants should set a good example. Slovenly attendants generally increase the number of dirty patients. The male attendants should not be permitted to wear loose holland frocks, which give them the appearance of butchers; and the female attendants should not be discouraged from observing the neatness and taste in dress which are natural to them. No mistake is greater than that of supposing that being dressed in unbecoming clothing, in stuff gowns and in mob-caps, is either a virtue in itself, or an incentive to virtue. Such sentiments form part of a gloomy and selfish system, including mortifications and degradations, especially unfavorable to goodness of any kind, and only gratifying to those who impose them. Such dresses are especially distasteful to English women of any class; they always discard these outward signs of poverty as soon as they are raised above the lowest condition of pauperism. A neglect of this really proper feeling is a frequent cause of discontent in asylums, and sometimes retards recovery.

Uniformity of dress is chiefly desirable as a check on escapes; but may in numerous cases among the female patients be wholly dispensed with. Many of the women should indeed be indulged in wearing neat articles of dress brought to them by their friends; there are even some whom it is impossible to soothe without this indulgence. As regards the male patients, uniformity of dress contributes greatly to their general good appearance, as a variety of male dress cannot be so neatly preserved as to avoid a miscellaneous shabbiness, from which female dresses, however cheap, are exempted by the care of the laundress. Good gray cloth, perhaps, preserves a decent appearance longer than cloth of any other colour, and it will bear frequent washing. Many of the men, on first admission, object to the round jacket worn at Hanwell; and certainly a short coat would be more becoming—its cost would only be a few additional shillings. Every male patient should be provided with a cotton neck-handkerchief of a dark colour, or a stock; and a straw hat or cap for the summer, and a black hat for the winter. A strong cotton forage-cap, grey or striped, the crown having a thick lining or light stuffing, to protect the head from the direct rays of the sun, is found very convenient. But it is best, in regard to the handkerchiefs, and the covering for the head, to allow the patients to choose that colour or kind which they prefer. Much comfort is imparted to many of the old and feeble male patients in the winter, by wearing a large cloth cape when out of doors; it is put on without trouble, and keeps the patient moderately warm, without impeding any kind of exercise.

It is scarcely necessary, I hope, to express my extreme disapprobation of dressing male pauper lunatics in poorer clothing than I have described, as in second-hand clothing which does not fit them, or in old leather breeches, and soldiers' jackets, dyed; excesses of economy which I have sometimes witnessed. In short, in regulating the dress of insane patients, as in every regulation for them, we must consider not only its first and indispensable uses, but its effects on the mind.

Our most intelligent male patients are always dressed with neatness, and are anxious to observe cleanliness in every respect. A suit of gray clothes taken care of by such patients, looks well even after six months' wear; and dresses so worn are still fit for wards in which the less intelligent patients are, who require frequent changes of clothing. Those who are employed in the farm and gardens, of course soil and wear out clothes sooner; but the average of suits of gray clothing supplied is one suit and a quarter per patient in a year, the cost of which is about twenty-three shillings. The average cost of the whole clothing of the patients is about one pound and fifteen shillings per annum per head.

Many private asylums are open to the charge of great neglect as respects the dress of patients of the classes far above pauperism. Tattered and threadbare coats, very shabby hats, trowsers not always free from an offensive smell; and equally slovenly dresses on the female side of the asylum, shoes out of repair, hair in curl-papers, make the unfortunate patients objects of pity or of ridicule. They feel themselves degraded, lose their self-respect, and with it the little self-control their malady has left them. It is very true, that in some cases the patients will not dress themselves properly, that they have an affection for old and ragged garments, and insist upon their being fit to go to court in, and are violently offended if better clothes are substituted for them ; but such cases form only a small proportion in any asylum; and in many instances, habits of personal neatness may long be preserved, and in some restored, after being long lost. Even an apparent disregard for cleanliness sometimes proves to have been the result of previous neglect and ill-treatment. Patients are often brought to Hanwell who are reported to us as uncleanly, but who do not prove so when properly attended to. Others who have been pronounced uncleanly, and sent to wards appropriated to such patients, have recovered the power of keeping themselves neat, and avoiding any uncleanly habits, after some accident has caused them to be subjected to the superintendence, and benefited by the care, of the attendants in the infirmaries. Such cases are not very frequent, but they prevent despair in circumstances which appear hopeless.

The rule should be, in private asylums, that each gentleman should be encouraged to dress according to his station, and to be at least as careful of his whole dress, his boots, his hat, his gloves, as he used to be when well. Ladies should not be allowed to forget that they are ladies; but should be required to dress appropriately, both in the morning and for dinner. Their friends are sometimes more in fault than they, and the patients are disfigured against their will; but it is disadvantageous to them to be thus permitted to fall into a negligence characteristic of advanced and incurable forms of disorder.

CHAPTER IV.

Diet of the Insane.—Its Influence on Recoveries, and on the Mortality of Asylums.—Hanwell Dietary.—Average weekly Cost of each Patient.— Employment of the Insane : its use and abuse.

DIET.—The quality, the quantity, the preparation, and the distribution of the diet of the patients in an asylum, is a subject in every way worthy of the careful consideration of the managers, the officers, and the attendants. The mere nutrition of the helpless, who cannot express their wants, or represent the most flagrant injustice and privation, demands all the care that humanity can suggest; but it is ordained that man should be capable of associating enjoyments with the mere partaking of food, which communicate satisfaction to the mind; and where the object is the restoration of mental tranquillity, attention to the diet, and its preparation and serving, rank among remedial measures, acting on the mind as well as on the body. All habitual physical discomfort is opposed to mental recovery, and a scanty, ill-cooked, unwholesome diet, creates a chronic uneasiness and dissatisfaction, impairs the health, and increases the mortality of an asylum. There is some reason to suppose that insane patients, shut within the bounds of an asylum, and necessarily leading a monotonous life, require, as prisoners are said to require, a greater quantity of food than persons do who are at large. It seems at all events to be established in asylums, that a very low diet conduces to a high mortality, and that the deaths diminish when the diet is improved—facts not difficult of belief, if we remember the number of feeble, paralytic, and phthisical patients in all asylums; and the number sinking from chronic and obscure disease, in all of whom life is capable of remarkable pro-

longation by careful management. Dr. Charlesworth is, perhaps, even right in considering insanity to be always a disease
of debility.   There are certainly, at all times, in all asylums,
many patients prone to sinking and death, in whom life is
only prolonged, and is visibly prolonged, by an extra allowance of diet, with the addition of porter and wine, and sometimes of brandy.   The insanity is itself, in certain classes, the
frequent result of half starvation, going on for years or for
generations.   The body has deteriorated, and the manifesta-
tions of the mind fail with the other functions. In some cases
the mere diet and general comfort of the asylum are sufficient,
first for relief, and ultimately for cure.   Patients who sit down
in dismal homes, to poor and ill-prepared food, and to very
little even of that, are unacquainted with the meaning of a
cheerful meal.   Their food is swallowed without pleasure ;
indigestion follows ; disordered conditions of the bowels ensue,
and physical and mental ills beyond the apothecary's stores
to cure.   Removed to an asylum, the sight of good food, in
sufficient quantity, surprises them ; they sit down to their
meals "free-minded and cheerfully-disposed,"—one of the
"sure 'precepts of long-lasting" enumerated by Lord Bacon ;
they soon become nourished ; the body and the mind recover
power ; and if we do not produce a cure, we produce content,
which is a great gain.

But the cures seem positively to be increased in number by
good diet.   Before the French Revolution, the diet at the
Bicêtre consisted, Pinel says, of a pound and a half of bread
daily.   This was given out in the morning, and instantly de-
voured, the rest of the day being passed in a kind of delirious
famine ; as travellers now report it to be by the patients in
the cages of the asylum at Cairo.   In 1791, the diet at the
Bicêtre was amended, the allowance of bread being increased
to two pounds, which was directed to be given in divided
portions, with some good soup, morning, noon, and evening.
The results of these changes are worthy of remembrance by
the directors and officers of public institutions, who are some-

times led into inhumanity, disguised as the respectable virtue
of economy. Under the old system, in 1784, out of 110 admissions there were 57 deaths. After the introduction of the
new system, the mortality on the total number admitted was
reduced to one eighth.

Dr. Thurnam, the excellent superintendent of the Retreat,
near York, has published a table in his late work on the
Statistics of Insanity, exhibiting the diet and the proportions
of recoveries, and of the mortality, in seven county asylums in
England. Although the recoveries in this table, being calculated on the admissions, cannot be strictly correct, their relative correctness is sufficient to illustrate the comparative effects
which it is his intention to show. He divides the asylums
into two groups : the first including those of Nottingham,
Stafford, and Gloucester ; the second those of Lancaster, the
West Riding of York, Suffolk, and Middlesex. This table was
constructed before certain improvements, which have now
taken place in the diet of the Middlesex and Lancaster Asylums, had been effected. In the first group, exclusive of
vegetables, the solid food, consisting of meat and cheese, and
of puddings, bread, and other farinaceous articles, amounted,
on an average, to 225 ounces per week. In the second group
it was only 150 ounces and a half. The proportion of recoveries and of deaths seems to have had some relation to these
differences ; the recoveries averaging 43·7 per cent. in the first
group, with the better diet, and only 36·75 in the second ;
and the mean mortality being, in the first group, 9·35 per
cent., and as high as 14·54 per cent. in the second. The
visiting justices made considerable additions to the diet at
Hanwell, in 1839, having required me, among my first duties,
to report upon it. Dr. Thurnam's table shows the satisfactory
results ; the proportion of the recoveries, still calculated on the
admissions, being, from 1831 to 1839, 22·12 ; and from 1839
to 1843, 28·75 ; and the mean annual mortality per cent.
being, before the improvement, 11·69, and afterward reduced
to 8·56. I must, however, observe, that the method of cal-

culating the recoveries on the admissions cannot but lead to
error. If the ultimate fate of every case admitted into an
asylum were accurately known, the comparison of the whole
number of recoveries with the whole number of admissions
would be simple and conclusive; but as this can never be accurately known, the number of admissions does not form a
just standard with which to compare the number of known
recoveries. If incurable cases are excluded from some asylums
and admitted into others, no calculation of cures ·on the admissions can justly show the curability of insanity in relation
to both; and the proportion of recoveries in one must seem
unduly greater than in the other. In any one year it is even
possible that the recoveries may exceed the admissions. But
the average daily number of patients in any asylum forms a
fixed standard, in relation to which the average of annual recoveries and deaths may be calculated with at least relative
accuracy; and with reference to asylums in which the regulations differ as to the kind of cases admitted.

In estimating the advantages of different asylums as places
of cure, the separate results furnish us, therefore, with no
accurate guidance. There is, I trust, no presumption in
saying that Hanwell ranks among the best conducted asylums. Yet its general proportion of cures is below that of
several others. But Hanwell is the refuge for all the worst
cases in Middlesex. Patients are neglected, or fastened down
and beaten, in numerous houses in the county, in the recent
state of malady, and when rendered intractable and dirty, are
sent to us to be cured. Or they are sent to us paralysed, aged,
bedridden, deprived of sense, covered with bruises or sores, to
die in our infirmaries. Of the first fifteen cases admitted at
Hanwell in 1846, one only was recent, or presented a slight
prospect of cure, and even this case was one in which the pre-
disposition to insanity was hereditary. We do not refuse admission to the epileptic, the paralysed, or the incurable. If
they do not recover, we do not send them away. This is their
place of rest; here they remain until they die. They conse-

quently fill up the places which might be occupied by the recent and the curable. This is inevitable in a county asylum for paupers only, and it ought not to be otherwise. It precludes our figuring in a table of comparative cures; but it makes our asylum the home and refuge of those who have no other earthly retreat. Of the recent cases, excluding the paralytic and epileptic, 50 per cent. are found to recover at Hanwell, being about the same number as in asylums where only recent cases are admitted, as Bethlem, St. Luke's, and Liverpool; always remembering, that of these 50, 25 may be considered as liable to relapse. In the article ' Lunatic Asylums,' in the ' Supplement to the Penny Cyclopædia,' there is a table, showing the mean number of the cures in the public asylums in the United Kingdom, for the last ten years, to have been 21·26 per cent. (See APPENDIX.)

There would also be some fallacy in ascribing these results, or approaches to them, wholly to an improved dietary. In all the asylums in the first group, patients of various classes are received, many above the condition of pauperism, and who are sent to the asylum not very long after the commencement of the attack. Moreover, a meager diet will usually be found the accompaniment of indifferent lodging, ill-ventilated bedrooms, scanty clothing, miserable shoes, bare heads, neglect of cleanliness, and a general treatment which makes the lunatic's condition "abject," to quote the well-selected term used by one of our intelligent male patients at Hanwell, who has had experience of the old treatment and the new. At Hanwell, at all events, the improved diet went hand in hand with improved lodging, better clothing, more careful ventilation of the wards, more systematic attention to the sick, an addition to the number of attendants, greater attention to the recreation of the patients, more care to abolish uncleanly wards, and, as the principle pervading all, the abolition of bodily fetters and restraints, and all the rude and violent accompaniments of the restraint system.

The diet of an asylum must in some degree be regulated by

the class of patients received into it, and, as Dr. Thurnam very properly observes, it should be for the insane pauper more liberal and nutritious than is usually found in his cottage, and for the wealthier patient simpler and plainer than that usual at his own table. Dr. Begley, one of the resident medical officers at Hanwell, has drawn up a table, showing the weekly allowance of solid and liquid food allowed to male patients in each county asylum in England. The quantity varies from 321 ounces of solid and 28 pints of fluid food, to 142 ounces of solid and 19½ pints of fluid food. In some of the Irish asylums scarcely any animal food is allowed; and with reference, it is to be presumed, to German patients, Dr. Jacobi recommends meat only twice or thrice a week; the diet on other days consisting of "broth of pearled barley, grits of rice, meal porridges made with water or milk, mulled beer, boiled fruits, easily-digested vegetables, puddings, &c." Much prudence is required in substituting the ordinary diet of any one country for another, and I feel sure that our English people generally require both animal food and beer to keep them in health in asylums.

At Hanwell the following is the present dietary, arranged, of course, entirely for pauper patients. It is neither scanty nor excessive. The weekly quantity of solid food for each male patient is two hundred and forty-seven and a half ounces, and of fluids fifteen pints; and although in different parts of the country the ordinary diet of the poor varies extremely, and renders modifications of diet in public institutions various, it is, perhaps, the best dietary for the pauper lunatics of England.

Breakfast.—The breakfast of the men consists of one pint of cocoa, with six ounces of bread; the women have the same quantity of cocoa and five ounces of bread. The cocoa has only recently been substituted for milk-porridge, to the great satisfaction of all the patients.

Dinner.—On Sundays, Tuesdays, Wednesdays, and Fridays, the dinner for each patient is five ounces of cooked meat, (seven ounces uncooked,) four ounces of yeast dumpling, and twelve ounces of vegetables. The meat is cooked by steam, except on Sundays, when it is baked, making the Sunday dinner a welcome variety. On Mondays the dinner consists of one pint of soup, with six ounces of bread; but as many patients dislike soup, eleven ounces of currant dumpling are occasionally substituted for it, and this seems to be approved of by the patients. On Thursdays, the dinner consists of twelve ounces of Irish stew, (containing an ounce and a half of cooked meat,) with six ounces of bread; and on Saturdays, of twelve ounces of meat-and-potato pie, containing about an ounce and a half of meat, two ounces being weighed out for each patient before cooking. Each patient has half a pint of beer at dinner time. In the fruit season, fruit pies are sometimes substituted for the meat pie on Saturday. Occasionally the patients have bacon and beans for dinner, and green vegetables are frequently substituted for potatoes. I believe all these varieties are as salutary as they are acceptable to the patients. The chief inconvenience of any fixed dietary is a want of variety; change of diet seeming to be desired, and even required, by patients of every class.

Tea.—The female patients alone are allowed tea in the afternoon; one pint of tea, with five ounces of bread, and half an ounce of butter, constituting at once their tea and supper. Many of the male patients feel the loss of their tea as a great privation when newly admitted. The friends of the patients are allowed to send them tea and sugar. The tea is prepared in the kitchen, by steam, and, probably from the extraction of the bitter principle of it, is not generally approved of; but in so large an asylum, making tea in the wards is scarcely practicable.

Supper.—The male patients have two ounces of cheese, six ounces of bread, and half a pint of beer, at seven in the evening.

Extras.—The men who work in the gardens, and on the farm, have half a pint of beer at eleven and at four o'clock,

and are also allowed one ounce of tea and four ounces of sugar
per week.   The women who work in the laundry are allowed
half a pint of beer at eleven o'clock, with bread and cheese.
The elderly and feeble women, in the ward No. 2, have a meat
dinner daily.   Those in the infirmaries, also, unless meat is
improper for them, have a daily meat dinner.   Fish or some
substitute for meat is allowed on Fridays, and in Lent, to the
Roman Catholic patients; and the sick have whatever the
medical officers think it right to order for them, and are supplied, during the night also, with tea, coffee, beef-tea, sago, and
arrow-root, with or without brandy, &c. &c.; and by these attentions they are kept fron sinking, and the tedious length of
the night hours is broken.

All this is effected at the expense of about eightpence a day
per patient, the actual cost of provisions for each being four
shillings and eightpence-halfpenny per week.   If it is gratifying to see what can be done for the comfort of insane patients
by this sum, it is also well to keep the amount itself in mind, as
there are seldom wanting unscrupulous persons who will undertake the whole charge of the insane for a sum scarcely exceeding it.   County asylums are consequently first much opposed,
and then opened with false expectations; and although everything is done for a time to realize such expectations, and always
at the expense of the patients, the delusion at length becomes
palpable, and the disappointment of the rate-payers extreme.
It may be useful, when speaking of this item of expenditure in
a county asylum, to mention that the average weekly expenditure for each patient in the Hanwell Asylum, for the quarter
ending March 31st, 1846, was, for provisions, four shillings
and eightpence-halfpenny; for house and bedding expenses,
one shilling and eightpence farthing; for salaries and wages
and maintenance of officers, attendants, and servants, one
shilling and eightpence three-farthings; for clothing, eightpence; for medicine and incidental expenses, threepence-half-
penny; the weekly total for each patient being nine shillings
and a penny; the annual total, twenty-three pounds, twelve
shillings and fourpence.

But it is not the mere quantity of food which alone contributes to the comfort of the meals of the patients at Hanwell. Its quality is most carefully attended to. The meat sent up to the wards is always of excellent quality; this and every other article of provisions or of stores being duly inspected by Mr. Clift, the storekeeper, who is actuated in the performance of his responsible duties, not only by a sense of what he undertakes to perform, but by a humane and lively interest in every detail that can contribute to the health and happiness of the patients. Those who inspect the asylum should never omit paying a visit to the storeroom, where they will find everything provided with an exactness and a solicitude worthy of this great establishment. An inspection of the farmyard, of the bakehouse, the brewhouse, and the kitchen will satisfy the intelligent spectator that the preparation of all the articles of food occupies the most vigilant attention of officers quite competent to the task of providing for so large a family. About 1080 persons are cooked for every day in the kitchen of the asylum; and its order, cleanliness, and tranquillity, at all hours, are the results of the very able superintendence of Mrs. Farrar, the housekeeper, now continued for sixteen years. He must be a fastidious person, who, with a healthy appetite, could not dine with satisfaction on the good, plain, well-prepared food, to be seen arranged in trays, on the long table in the kitchen at Hanwell, every day at one o'clock. Precisely at that hour, a bell is rung, and two patients with one attendant come from each male ward, and carry away the tray, and the beer-cans belonging to it. The dinners for all the female wards are sent to the female side of the asylum a quarter of an hour earlier, and then distributed through the wards in the same manner. As soon as these are received into the several wards, the meat is divided into portions, the vegetables and dumplings placed with each patient's portion, good and hot gravy is poured into each plate, salt is placed within everybody's reach, and the allowance of beer is poured out. Whilst

4

all this is doing, the patients remain in the gallery, and they only come into the day-room or dining-room of their ward when all is announced to be ready. They then find each patient's dinner set out for him on a table covered with a decent tablecloth, and all in perfect order. The attendants see that each patient takes his seat so as not to incommode his neighbours, preventing crowding in one place, and wide spaces being left in other places, without which attention discontent is occasioned, and quarrels may arise. As the attendants do not dine with the patients, they have nothing to do but to attend to them, and to keep order. In the male wards at Hanwell all this is done systematically ; but either greater difficulty exists or less care is taken on the female side of the house. The male patients take more pains to keep the plates, knives, forks, and beer-tins clean, and sit down to dinner with far more order than the women. All stand up for a few moments, their heads uncovered, whilst a grace is read by one of themselves, at the head of the table ; many respond "Amen!" and then they sit down with a cheerfulness which it is gratifying to witness. What still more strongly exemplifies the order that may be introduced among the insane is, that in the male refractory wards the same regulations are carried into effect, and I have even observed the patients in one of them sitting quietly after their dinner was concluded, and only quitting the table when thanks had been given in a short grace, read, as at the commencement of the dinner, by a patient.

Punctuality as to time, cleanliness in all that appertains to the tables, an equal and careful division of the food and beer into portions, order in sitting down, are matters of great consequence to the general comfort of the patients, and when properly attended to, contribute to relieve their distress on first admission. A well educated female patient told me that she was, thirty years ago, first sent to a large asylum near London, and that the impression made on her mind by the mode in which the meals were conducted was, that she had been sentenced to live among cannibals. The desirable order now described can only be obtained by means of good attendants, well instructed in their duty, and diligently overlooked by resident officers, who should very frequently visit the wards at the dinner, and breakfast, and supper hours, without which vigilance the tendency to slovenliness is sure to show itself again after a time. These particulars form almost daily objects of attention with Dr. Begley and Dr. Hitchman, the resident medical officers of the asylum; and this attention is found to be necessary for the perpetuation of observances, of which the use is not always generally obvious to those from whom they are required.

All the patients at Hanwell, who can sit at table, use knives and forks, if capable of holding them in their hands. Patients who are violently excited, or too infirm to cut their meat, have their dinners taken to them by one of the attendants, with a spoon, instead of a knife and fork; the meat, vegetables, and dumplings being first cut into proper-sized pieces. Those who are sick, and in bed, are very carefully attended to in this respect, and it is not unusual to see one of the other patients volunteering to stay by the bedside of the sick until they have dined. Knives are, of course, occasionally withheld from the suicidal; but occasionally only. The plates are usually of metal; but crockery has been lately introduced into some of the wards, and the breakage is very insignificant. The knife is only sharpened along a portion of its edge, and the fork has very short prongs. For the fork, however, so long in use, and of which the shape is most inconvenient as well as unsightly, whilst it really presents no security, a fork of nickel has recently been substituted in several of the wards, shaped like an ordinary silver fork. Its appearance is much better; it is lighter and more convenient for use; it is not more expensive than the old fork, and, in my opinion, it is actually safer. When the patients are all kindly and properly treated, and their meals are comfortable, and the attendants do not neglect the order and arrangement which have been mentioned, there will be found very little disposition in the patients to employ the knives and forks as offensive weapons; they put them to a better use.

If all these arrangements are thought to be necessary, and found to be useful, in an asylum only containing pauper lunatics, how necessary and how useful they must be in asylums containing patients of a higher class will readily be concluded. It is impossible to be too careful in directing that all the service of the table should be in accordance with the habits of the patients. The sense of banishment from home, and of confinement, and the consciousness of mental infirmity and dependence, are mitigated in the mind of many a silent, uncomplaining patient by these means. All the comforts added of late years, and with so much advantage, to the wards of county asylums—such as movable tables and chairs, window-blinds, plants, musical instruments, bagatelle boards, books, and pictures, with free access to agreeable gardens—show that the majority of the insane of any class are inclined to respect the decent arrangements made for them; and it will generally be found that the more conformable the furniture of the rooms, the tables, &c., of the higher class of the insane is to their habits and rank, the less they will be disposed to destroy or derange it. During violent paroxysms of mania, they are of course regardless of everything; and everything about them should be plain, simple, and secure. But when convalescence begins it should be respected. Among the depressing recollections of the insane of the higher classes, when recovering from insanity, I know that none are more frequent, or felt to be more degrading, than those connected with any want of respect shown to them, or any disregard of decent customs as to their meals. Yet, without great attention, they will sometimes be found, when quite well enough to appreciate what is done, sitting down to a dinner of meat, vegetables, and pudding, all sent to them on one plate. Negligences of this kind produce fretfulness and discontent, and tend to retard convalescence. If attendants are allowed to practise this kind of negligence, they soon fall into habits of rudeness, and even of inhumanity, fancying that the patients do not observe their conduct, and that their feelings are of no consequence.

It is, in general, quite unnecessary that there should be anything peculiar in the shape of the knives and forks used by patients of this class, when they are neither violent nor determinedly suicidal. At the Retreat at York, where the knives and forks guarded as I have described were first employed, ordinary knives and forks have now been long in use; and the same is the case at the asylums of Heidelburgh and Pirna. The richer patients at Siegburg have stone-china coffee and tea pots, use glasses, &c. In the asylum at Utica, New York, Dr. Brigham reports that all the patients use " knives and forks, tumblers, and handsome table crockery." In some English private asylums, silver knives are preferred for patients thought likely to make any improper use of knives that are sharper. Whatever is used at table, it is of the first importance that it should be scrupulously clean ; and all the meals should be ready at precise hours. Great regularity of hours tends much to break the monotony of private as well as of public asylums, and should be strictly attended to. Everything should be performed or ready at the appointed hour, and the tediousness of waiting entirely unknown, as it always leads to complaints and irregularities.

Employment.—Among the means of relieving patients from the monotony of an asylum, and of preserving the bodily health, and, at the same time, of improving the condition of the mind, and promoting recovery, employment of some kind or other ranks the highest. Its regulation is proportionably important. The spirit in which it is conducted should be conformable to the general spirit of the asylum; and its abuse should be carefully guarded against. A few years ago the idea of entrusting patients with various tools and implements, or even of occupying them, except to a very limited extent, was only entertained at Hanwell, among the large asylums near London. It was introduced at Hanwell, from Wakefield, by the late Sir William Ellis. But workshops have lately

been erected at Bethlem; and, as regards county asylums, there
is now a great disposition in the officers to set every patient to
work as soon as admitted; sometimes very improperly, and
when, perhaps, work has made the poor creature mad. A man
just admitted is perhaps sent off to the shoemaker's shop before
his case can have been considered by the physician; and a
poor melancholy woman, or a frightened, agitated girl is set
to work immediately with a needle and thread, to pursue, as
if in a mere workhouse, the same sedentary occupation which
has already destroyed her health.   There is, however, a
difficulty in persuading a shoemaker or tailor to work at any
occupation but his own.   The tailors, especially, are so averse
to locomotion, that when a new and better workshop was made
for them at Hanwell, in 1841, it was not easy at first to per-
suade them to walk across the kitchen-yard to it. Sempstresses
also have usually been so long accustomed to live without
exercise and fresh air, that they are quite contented to sew
from morning to night.   In vain does the physician, day by
day, represent the evil of this, and try to induce the proper
attendants to take them out.   The workrooms, storerooms, and
other parts of the building where patients are employed, at
Hanwell, are particularly large and airy, and the health of the
patients cannot be said to be extensively injured by any even
of the in-door occupations; but the medical care of an asylum
is incomplete which leaves a crowd of persons in a heated
room all the day, except at meal times; and in some of the
younger and recent and curable cases, the prescriptions of
the physician are baffled by the neglect of his advice that the
patients should take exercise.   This is one of numerous instances illustrating the great disadvantage of having any
officers in an asylum empowered to act without the physician's
sanction.   The regulation of the employment of the patients
is the regulation of a highly important remedy, and should
never be attempted without his assistance.   No patient recently admitted should be employed at all, until the physician
has first put the patient's name in a list kept for the purpose,

specifying the kind of work most desirable. In many cases of recent mania and melancholia, work is positively detrimental to the patient ; and in chronic cases it is sometimes much objected to, and becomes, on that account,· useless, if not hurtful. Generally speaking, sedentary occupations appear to be less favorable to the recovery of our patients at Hanwell than active occupations. More women get well who are employed in the kitchens, laundries, and wards than in the workrooms; and more men recover who work in the gardens and on the farms than in the tailors' or the shoemakers' shops.

Farm and garden work is not only more active, but more various, and therefore more remedial. This advantage, and that of its being carried on in the open air, and exciting no violent emotions, are justly enumerated amongst its recommendations by Dr. Jacobi: but I do not think that the occupation of a farmer so little disposes to mental derangement as he considers it to do. Dr. Parry observed that the slow riding about of farmers when superintending their workmen, and other circumstances, strongly disposed them to determinations to the head, to which their general mode of living may readily be supposed to contribute ; and this state of the circulation not unfrequently becomes associated with mania or melancholy.

A wish, laudable in itself, to make the labour of the patients profitable, leads, no doubt, to the general employment of patients in their own trades; but this, for a tailor, or for a shoemaker, or a weaver, or a dressmaker, is often the worst thing that can be done, and takes away the chance of recovery. An occasional change of the kind of work is sometimes seen to be serviceable ; and I have so repeatedly noticed the cheerfulness diffused among the female patients by employment in the season for fresh fruit and vegetables, when more help is required in the kitchen, as to wish that occasional and various employment could be devised for many who are fretful when not employed. It is probably with some view of this kind that Dr. Jacobi proposes, that in the winter season the sedentary or imbecile should be provided with baskets of beans, peas, &c., mixed together, and to be separated by them. I fear this occupation would be found rather unprofitable; but that there are many patients capable of some employment, who are sedentary and becoming imbecile, I cannot doubt. When knitting was introduced among the female patients at Hanwell, a few years ago, I noticed that some of this class of patients were employed for the first time since I had known them.

Constant and regular work cannot properly be exacted from insane persons; and they should not be kept at work so many hours as sane people. Those patients who are employed in the workshops, laundries, bakehouses, &c., should be induced occasionally to walk round the field or gardens; and there can be no good reason for making the work a constant excuse for keeping away the patients from morning and evening prayers. Forcing the patients to work against their will, compelling them to one kind of work when they prefer another, and prohibiting the employment which they prefer; as well as the use of threats, the limitation of their diet, and recourse to devices for mortifying the patients who are indisposed to work, are faults not often, I hope, committed in asylums; but they are not unknown, and they are of a nature to be overlooked in the pride of a long list of patients employed. In general, there is no want of a disposition to be occupied in those capable of exertion, and many patients are wretched if not allowed to work. To stigmatize as indolence what is the mere result of a malady which immediately reduces the nervous energy, and is often the beginning of paralysis, is an error into which no medical man would fall, and from which his opinion ought to protect any of his patients. There are some who are really indolent, but few of them who may not be in some way or other encouraged to some kind of occupation. I do not speak of punishments for those who are disinclined to work, believing that such are never inflicted on the insane in this country; but they appear to be practised in some of the asylums of the Continent; and some vigilance is required to prevent a similar abuse creeping into all large asylums, and, I believe, especially in the female workrooms.

In the last Annual Report of Hanwell, it is shown, that of 418 male patients then in the asylum, 219 were employed. Of these, 75 were occupied in the gardens, or on the farm, and 40 as helpers in the wards. We have a carpenter's shop, an upholstery room, a tailor's shop, and shoemaker's shop, and tinman's shop. Some are employed in attending the painters, bricklayers, or whitewashers; some in the engine-house, the smith's shop, or the gas-house; several in occasional work; and four or five in the printing-office.

Of 567 women, 314 were employed, of whom 69 were in the laundry, and 49 were helpers in the wards; 18 were in the kitchen and dairy, and as many as 178 were employed in needlework.

The quantity of work thus done is considerable. All the clothing of the patients (except the shoes) and all the bedding is entirely made up in the asylum; all the washing of the immense establishment is performed in the laundries; and all the mending in the wards and workrooms. Vegetables are cultivated for the use of the asylum. Carpenter's work is carried on to a great extent; the bed-frames, rocking-horses, tables, arm-chairs, benches, &c., being made within the asylum. It is obvious that a great variety of employment might yet be introduced; but there is difficulty in introducing such as would pay the expenses of the materials used, and the superintendence required; for the work-masters must exercise as much vigilance over those employed under them as the attendants do in the wards; and if new employments are resorted to, more work-masters must be engaged, capable, not only of directing the work, but of teaching those to work who have had little or no previous instruction. In this respect, the master-workmen have not yet shown any zeal, although I am quite satisfied, that among our younger male patients, especially among the epileptic, and even among those who are accounted imbecile, there are some who might be taught useful work, with

4 §

an increase of their happiness, and some benefit to their minds.

Many of the incurable patients work so steadily and tranquilly, and many of the convalescent are capable of regular employment so long before they are altogether fit to take care of themselves, that it is impossible not to wish to see some establishments founded, intermediate between asylums and ordinary life, in which profitable labour could be supplied to some for a short time, and to others for a longer period. Such establishments would become houses of cure ; and if arrangements could be made in them for the temporary care of the poor neglected children of the insane, much future evil might be kept from their families, and much distress of mind removed from the patients themselves. In those asylums to which a charitable fund is attached, this project deserves serious consideration. A mere donation to a patient discharged recovered is liable to be taken advantage of by the parish. What is wanted is the means of placing the patient and his family in a position favorable to resuming a course of successful industry, which cannot be done by a penniless man who finds his children in the workhouse, and is without any means of giving them a home.

I do not know that any systematic attempts have been made to introduce work among patients in England of a higher class than mechanics. Ladies are seldom without some resources of this kind, which, indeed, never seem to fail them until the mind has become very greatly enfeebled. One might imagine many gentlemen when insane deriving solace from turning, making nets, light carpenter's work, gardening, &c.

CHAPTER V.

Attendants, Appointment and Qualifications of.—Their daily Duties.—
Arrangements for Night-watching in an Asylum.

AN indispensable condition for protecting and controlling the insane, without having recourse to bodily restraints, is the command of the services of a sufficient number of efficient attendants. In public asylums for the poor, the proportion of attendants is about one attendant to seventeen patients. One to fifteen would be better; but by giving one to thirteen in the more troublesome wards, and one to twenty or more in the quiet wards, the proportion of one to seventeen for the whole asylum may suffice. In the French asylums, the proportion is one to ten; but the attendants have other duties than those immediately relative to the patients, which makes several of them nearly useless. In private asylums for patients of the richer classes, the proportion should be one to five, or one to three; or, in particular cases, one to two.

If I may rely on my own observation, no subject connected with the management of the insane, either in asylums or in private practice, has received less adequate attention than the selection of proper attendants, their proper treatment, their just government, and their instruction in the various, and peculiar, and exhausting duties which necessarily devolve upon them. The important and delicate task of regulating the conduct of persons of unsound mind, of controlling excitement, restraining waywardness, or removing mental depression, is unavoidably confided to persons of limited education; but these are too frequently chosen with little regard to their disposition, temper, or intelligence: they are permitted to commence their duties with as little preparation as if their office

was merely that of a servant, and are governed either with
severity and injustice, or without the consideration and indulgence requisite to support their patience, and to encourage
them to be considerate and indulgent to those on whom they
attend, and who are wholly in their power.

The idea of the attendants being selected without reference
to the medical superintendent of an asylum is so extremely
absurd, that nothing but its being entertained and acted upon
by the governing bodies of asylums would suggest any allusion
to it. The patients of any asylum in which this regulation
prevails are generally deprived of the principal means of recovery, for the attendants are at the head of the remedial
means employed by the physician. To compel him to treat
his patients with the aid of attendants in whom he can have
very little confidence, and for whose fidelity, or even for whose
kindness, he has no security, is as injudicious as it would be to
oblige him to employ drugs of an inferior quality, selected by
persons unacquainted with the articles of the materia medica.
In private practice the absurdity of the plan becomes immediately evident ; the custom in asylums being tantamount to
having an attendant for a private gentleman selected by the
neighbouring gentry (a sort of committee), or by his housekeeper (a kind of matron), and not by his physician. Of all
the physician's remedial means, they are the most continually
in action: all that cannot be done by his personal exertion depends upon them. The character of particular patients, and
of all the patients of a ward, takes its colour from the character of the attendants placed in it. On their being proper or
improper instruments—well or ill-trained — well or ill-dis-
ciplined—well or ill-cared for,—it depends whether many of
his patients shall be cured or not cured; whether some shall
live or die; whether frightful accidents, an increased mortality,
incalculable uneasiness and suffering, and occasional suicides,
shall take place or not. Painful, therefore, is the situation of
the physician to an asylum who is liable, at every visit, to
find forty or fifty of his patients put under the care of new at-

tendants; separated from those to whom they were attached, and who had become acquainted with their peculiarities; and subjected to the rude dominion either of attendants without experience, and whom he sees at once to be without capacity for the duties he requires of them, or, what is worse, of attendants trained in asylums where the system of restraint is in full operation, and who are consequently versed in all the neglect, the harshness, and the concealment which can inflict suffering on the patients, and which must cause disappointment of all his designs.

The occasional acquisition, under such a system, of a good attendant, is merely a happy accident; and the physician can even then never feel sure that the attendant will be allowed to remain. Sometimes attendants will be discharged for faults which the physician would occasionally pardon in those from whom so much is expected; and sometimes they will be retained when he knows them to be unworthy of trust, or even guilty of cruelty. No attendant should, in short, be appointed or dismissed without reference to the physician, and his full approval. His experience teaches him alone all the qualifications indispensably required of them.

As a general rule, the attendants, when entering on their duties, should not be more than thirty years of age, or rather, five and twenty. Male attendants, who are older, if they have been in the army, or accustomed to responsibility, often prove valuable; but I have scarcely ever known a female attendant prove efficient who commenced her duties after thirty, and some of the best whom I have known, and whom many years of trial have now proved, began their duties before they were twenty. Activity and good spirits are required, and these qualities do not increase with years. The temper of older persons unaccustomed to the insane is easily ruffled; they have often been depressed by the events of life, and either give way to the oppressive influences of an asylum, or try to keep up their energies by stimulants. This is particularly the case with female attendants who enter late on such duties;

and altogether—and putting humanity as much out of the question as it generally is where attendants are selected in the manner I have mentioned—there is no cherished fallacy greater than that of supposing that plain, middle-aged, ill-dressed women are more moral, or more orderly in their habits and life, than young, active, well-dressed nurses. The best attendants, both male and female, are to be found in the class of persons who are qualified to be upper servants, and their services may always be commanded in an asylum where a fair remuneration and a prospect of comfort are held out to them.

But the first requisite for an attendant, if conjoined with a moderate share of understanding, is benevolence. I fear this is a quality often wholly omitted in the inquiry into the character of attendants. Certainly, many have been observed by me in such situations, and entrusted with the care of private patients, whose physiognomy and whose voices proclaimed at once their want of such a quality; men chosen apparently on account of their possessing the frame of a prize-fighter, and sharp-tempered women, with merely capacity enough to be under-housemaids. Yet these attendants constantly live with the patients, and must be entirely relied upon for the performance of the various duties which are presently to be mentioned. There is generally, of course, in asylums, a rapid succession of attendants so ill qualified as these; and sometimes for a whole year, or for successive years, some particular wards are thus kept continually unsettled and ill-managed. Irregularities, accidents, injuries, and confusion then present themselves daily to the physician's observation, and he is powerless to remove them. It cannot be concealed or denied that where such regulations prevail, and such attendants are appointed, the patients have not all the advantages which the public have a right to expect should be extended to them, and that a great duty is neglected. The great object of establishing and perpetuating a system of kindness, which nothing can disturb, and which generates the confidence of the patients, and acts as the most powerful and salutary of all restraints, is thus defeated.

It is quite impossible for me to convey to the reader a just idea of the mischievous cruelty exercised in private houses, where single patients are intrusted to attendants supplied from private asylums in which restraints are permitted to be used. They invariably arrive armed with a strait waistcoat; they almost invariably put it on the patient, whose subsequent violence becomes an excuse for drawing it closer and tighter, until the skin is ulcerated. The legs are then fastened, and the legs and back become ulcerated also. Cleanliness is then disregarded; food is refused in some instances after such degrading treatment, and death, I sincerely believe, is an occasional result.

The duties of an attendant in an asylum begin early in the morning, are incessant during the day, and end late. The visitors who are merely attended by them through the wards, and see them neatly dressed, and apparently at leisure to answer every curious or every idle question, can by no means appreciate the labour necessary to produce the cleanliness, or the continued watchfulness required to maintain the order, which are generally so much the objects of admiration in the wards of such institutions. The regulation of their daily duties at Hanwell is perhaps as useful as any of which any account can be easily referred to ; but its adaptation to asylums in other parts of the country, or in other countries, must be regulated by the judgment of different superintendents. Habits of life and climate are the principal circumstances necessarily modifying such arrangements.

At six o'clock, a.m., they are expected to unlock the doors of the patients' bedrooms ; most of the patients being wearied with ten hours passed in bed, or in solitude, and anxious for liberty. A few patients, unfit to be at large, cannot be let out so early, or until the attendants have time, after attending to the washing and combing, and to the breakfasts of the other patients, to pay them the especial attention which they

require. Until lately, the insane were not more favorably
situated as regarded the means of preserving personal cleanliness than the soldier in barracks ; but lavatories, fitted up in
the manner already described, are now attached to almost
every ward at Hanwell, and the attendants can more easily
perform the required duty of ascertaining the state of the skin
of each patient, so as to report any soreness, discoloration, or
other change, to the resident medical officers, at the morning
visit, together with the state of health of any particular patient, or anything altered in the state of the appetite, or remarkable in the evacuations, or any other accident.   Without
this observation, some feeble patients may sink day by day
almost unnoticed, whom timely attention will revive.   Medicines are frequently to be given, or baths administered, early
in the morning, and it is very essential that this should not be
omitted when ordered.

Soon after getting up, or at half-past six, the female patients
who are employed in the laundry are to be collected and taken
thither by the laundrymaids ; but this duty will be done by
the laundrymaids in a very rude and irregular manner unless
some of the assistant female officers are stirring in the wards
at that hour.   Patients who object to going to the laundry
will sometimes be forced to go against their will, although
their disinclination may arise from a feeling of weariness or
exhaustion. The importance of the duties of the laundry being
regularly performed may be productive of some disposition to
overwork the patients employed in it ; but when any patient
strongly objects to going, the case should be referred to the
medical officers.

At seven, a.m., the attendants ought to go to the kitchen, or
wherever the distribution can most conveniently be made, for
the bread, butter, &c., required for the patients of each ward
during the day.   The punctual and orderly performance of
this duty wholly depends on the regularity of the housekeeper, whose representations as to any departure from order
and punctuality should always meet with immediate attention.

At this hour also, any attendant who has had leave of absence for the night is expected to be in the wards; but if eight were the hour for this appearance, it would be much more easily and much better attended to, nor would any particular inconvenience arise from the alteration, and the attendant would still be ready to go to chapel, or to attend to the breakfasts of the patients. Each ward having at least two attendants attached to it, the patients are never supposed to be left unattended.

Morning prayers, occupying about a quarter of an hour, are read in the chapel at Hanwell at eight o'clock, before the patients have breakfasted. Nine o'clock would be a preferable hour, as by that time both patients and attendants would have breakfasted, and be readier to attend. The hour would also be more convenient to the chaplain, who is not usually a resident officer in asylums; and it would also deprive the other officers of any reasonable excuse for not attending. Between two and three hundred patients usually assemble in the chapel at the morning and afternoon services on Sunday, and about half the number in the mornings and evenings of week days. It is therefore expected that not fewer than five female and four male attendants should accompany the patients to chapel; and in my own opinion every officer of an asylum, not especially prevented, and all the members of their families, and their servants should also attend. The effect of this on the patients would be very satisfactory, and the attendants would be encouraged, by example, not to slide into negligence as to collecting the patients, and attending to their dress and behaviour in chapel. Merely requiring a numerical list of those who attend leads to deception; and if there is service at all, it ought to command the respectful observance of all the residents in the asylum every day in the week.

The patients at Hanwell breakfast as soon as the morning prayers are concluded. This meal ought to be frequently superintended by assistant officers, and great care should be taken that those patients who are yet left in their bedrooms are not forgotten. The breakfast of such patients should also be taken to them by an attendant, and not by other patients.

As soon as the breakfast is concluded, the more active duties of the ward-attendants must commence. Every bed-room has to be cleaned out, and all the galleries and day-rooms are to be made neat. The bed-frames and, in many cases, the bedding, various articles of clothing, and in asylums where straw is used, all the straw, and everything uncleanly or broken, and all accumulations of litter and rubbish, must be diligently removed. Every window must now be opened, in almost all weathers, at least for a time; many windows have of course been opened long before, or, in the summer season, all the night. In warm and dry weather, it is even unnecessary, in many cases, to shut the windows during the night, especially in the dormitories; and if the shutters of the bedrooms in the refractory wards are closed, the windows ought certainly to be left open, to prevent the irritability of the patients being very much increased. The attendants ought thoroughly to understand that no excuses will ever be admitted for uncleanliness, or for any bad smell, in any part of the asylum; and that if the floors require daily washing they must be dried as quickly as possible; and no pails, or mops, or brushes, or gas-keys, or steps, or any mischievous moveable thing, be left in the way of the patients. Many accidents are thus avoided; to prevent which restraints were formerly much and very needlessly employed.

A partial and very convenient clearing of the wards may be effected at the time these active occupations commence, by the male patients who are employed out of doors, or in the shops, and the female patients who are employed in the workrooms, being now collected by the superintendents of the different kinds of employment, and taken away to their occupations. The duty of collecting them should be performed in an orderly, tranquil, and encouraging manner. Of the patients not employed out of the wards, some remain, and materially assist the attendants in their heaviest work; others get out at once into the airing-courts.

At half-past nine, or ten, at the latest, the infirmaries, and the sick in all the wards, should be made ready for the morning medical visit. The sick diet-lists, made out every day, should be ready for inspection or alteration in each infirmary; and everything required for the sick for the day, as far as can then be foreseen, should be ordered in writing. An attendant from each infirmary, or, what is better, a head attendant from each side of the asylum, should take the lists and orders at once to the store-rooms and kitchen, accompanied by two or three patients, and the wine, porter, broth, or other extras, should be there immediately delivered to them, or at the time for which any order is given.

All the wards should now be visited, not only by the medical officers, but by those to whom the order and cleanliness of the wards and the domestic superintendence of the attendants is especially intrusted. It is from their care that the medical officers have to expect that neatness and cleanliness everywhere prevail; and at this hour the whole house should be ready for inspection, and all the attendants should be neatly dressed. This is the department of the matron and steward, and their assistants. After this time, no patients should be found in their bedrooms, except those who are sick or very feeble, or are too much excited to be interfered with. Attempts should be made to get every patient up; and those who are excited and negligent of cleanliness should be moved out of one bedroom to another, to permit the room in which they have slept to be cleaned. Unless very much excited, the patient should be dressed and taken out. As soon as possible after this time—not later than eleven in temperate weather, earlier in summer, and about noon in winter—every patient who can walk should be taken out of doors, or persuaded to walk about, one of the attendants of each ward always going with them. A very violent patient, if permitted to walk about, should have an attendant on each side of him, and they should endeavour to keep him in good humour. Very few are so violent as not to be benefited by being out for a short time every day.

It is now that the various condition of those under their charge requires the various appliances or substitutes for mechanical restraints during the day, which the attendants have been taught to avail themselves of. The most troublesome of the patients, when no restraints are used, are not to be left in their rooms, neglected and forgotten; the bed, and sometimes the room also, must be changed: fresh air must be admitted, comfortable food administered, the patients must be washed, or have a warm bath, and then have clean clothing put on. Those who tear their clothing must have it made of ticking, or some other strong material; those who undress themselves must have their clothes fastened by small locks instead of buttons, patterns of all which may be seen at Hanwell. Those who are very violent and frantic must be placed in the padded rooms, and reported to the medical officers; as also those who are sick and feeble. In every case where these reasons against it do not exist, the patients must be taken out for exercise: even violent patients must not always be kept shut up in small rooms, but be allowed to walk where they can do no mischief, or accompanied by one or two attendants. There are few patients so violent as not by degrees to be calmed by these daily attentions; scarcely any so surly as not to be soothed by them. Excitement may continue long, or often recur; but the patient will seldom be fierce or revengeful, or quite insensible to the attendant's care and kindness.

At eleven o'clock, when the patients who are active and tolerably well are out of doors, walking, or occupied with amusements partaken of by the attendants; some in the airing-courts, and all the quietest and best behaved in the larger fields or grounds, the boundaries being carefully watched, and all the ground vigilantly overlooked by the attendants; the other patients, those at work, for instance, and those in the house, and disabled from work or from walking, are variously attended to. The out-door workers have beer, and the women employed in the laundry have beer and bread and cheese; and the feeble and sick have some excellent broth, or porter, or wine; and the due administration of these refreshments is a duty which ought to be most scrupulously performed by the attendants, and in many cases superintended by assistant officers.

Considerable difficulty is always found in effecting a proper superintendence of the patients in the grounds; and it never can be effected unless some of the officers are frequently to be seen there. No time is more favorable for conversing with several of the patients than when they are walking about; and if the officers never go into the exercising-grounds the attendants are naturally inclined to conclude that this part of their own duty is also of little consequence, and the patients are allowed to wander about, to quarrel, dispute, or come to blows, or to escape over the fences, or to lie in the heat of the sun, or on the damp grass. These things call for the continual exercise of the attention, both of attendants and officers. There is no time in the day in which the attendants can be said to have nothing to do. The inattention of a few minutes, and the neglect of some ordinary and common precaution, may be the cause of occurrences of the most lamentable kind.

The most convenient dinner hour for the patients in an asylum not intended for the richer classes is one. An hour before that time (or at twelve o'clock), the attendants should take the trays, beer-cans, and dishes to the kitchen, or wherever the distribution of the dinners and the beer takes place. In this, as in everything in which patients can be properly engaged, they are assisted by them, and also in carrying the dinners, &c., at one o'clock, from the kitchen to the different wards. This duty always seems to be a pleasant one to the patients, and is performed with much alacrity and cheerfulness, and it scarcely ever happens that they are interrupted in it by the patients of any of the wards through which they have to pass.

When speaking of the diet of asylums, the attentions required from the attendants during the dinner-hour of the patients were particularly mentioned. By such attentions all accidents and ill behaviour may generally be prevented. Those who visit the male wards at Hanwell at dinner-time, may see, in different day-rooms or galleries, from thirty to fifty insane persons sitting down to dinner, with quite as much order as so many sane labourers ; but this gratifying effect is produced by systematic and constant care to provide them with good food, equally distributed, and comfortably served ; and by their having sufficient space, and every attempt at irregularity being prevented by timely admonition, or, if required, the timely removal of the disorderly. It is most desirable that the officers of an asylum should manifest the interest they take in a meal so essential to the comfort of the patients, by frequently visiting the wards at such times ; their presence seems always to give satisfaction to the patients, and it also prevents some negligences, especially as regards the sick or those not dining at the table with the rest. The attendants are generally too much inclined to delegate the duty of carrying the dinner and beer of such patients to some other patient ; but this ought by no means to be allowed. Without frequent superintendence, also, such patients will have their dinners taken to them without knife or fork, or spoon, or salt ; and the habit of attending to all these points should be strictly kept up. Carelessness as to individual patients soon leads to general negligence ; general discomfort follows, and the proper character of an asylum, and a proper influence on the habitual feelings of the patients, cannot be maintained. The greatest results desired in an asylum depend very much upon very small attentions, perpetually exercised.

Among the patients most severely affected, some may have a repugnance for food ; some may refuse it in consequence of thinking it poisoned; and some from mere obstinacy. These cases require a discriminating attention: every such case should be reported to the medical officers. In recent attacks aversion to food is a common symptom; but it does not, generally, last many days. Some patients experience a like aversion to food in every recurrent paroxysm. The feeble and sinking are often unable to take food, or to digest it if taken. A disordered condition of the stomach frequently exists, in which food is most distasteful to the patient, who even considers it to be poisoned. All these are cases requiring careful medical attention. When refusal to take food arises from some obstinate delusion or a disposition to self-destruction, kind treatment, varied food, and patient persuasion will often overcome what appears a formidable difficulty. Some patients will abstain from food for a few days, and then eat voraciously. The attendants must make themselves acquainted with all these eccentricities of particular patients. For more than four years it has not been found necessary at Hanwell, in any case, to administer food by force; although we have during all that time always had nearly a thousand patients in the asylum.

An hour is allowed for the dinner of the patients, and by two o'clock everything is removed from the tables; the floors of the dining-rooms are swept, some of the patients are employed in cleaning all the dinner utensils; the patients return to the workshops or workrooms in which they are employed, or to the garden and farm, the superintendents of which have already dined; and the ward-attendants have themselves leisure to dine. I think it most important to the comfort of the attendants that they should have a dining-room on each side of the asylum, separate from the wards, and that one half of them should dine at two o'clock, and the other half at half-past two. If they have conscientiously performed the duties of the preceding seven hours, they have well earned the half-hour's relief from the wards thus obtained. Their dining-room ought, in every respect, to be a pattern of neatness; a head attendant should be charged with keeping proper order in it; and their dinners ought to be good and carefully sent up. Whatever dissatisfies attendants entails some evil consequences on the patients; and if they are expected to be good-humoured and forbearing, they must be made reasonably comfortable. The plan of requiring them to dine in the wards, at the same table with the numerous patients for whom they have carved, is quite inconsistent with their comfort, or even with their health. They are heated and wearied, and cannot eat their dinner in such circumstances; it is therefore put by for an irregular meal at some irregular hour, and the neglect of some daily duty or other is the general consequence.

During the dinner-hour of the attendants, no ward should be left entirely without an attendant; and at five minutes after three o'clock all the attendants should again be in the wards. Soon afterward, if the weather is dry and not too hot, the patients should be out of doors again, in the airing-courts or the grounds; and they should remain out from an hour to two hours, discretion being used in regard to particular patients in different seasons of the year, and also to their various inclinations, but with a constant endeavour to promote some activity in all. In the summer, the great heat of the afternoon is unfavorable to the patients; but in such seasons they should always be out of doors for an hour or an hour and a half before their bedtime; as by this an opportunity is afforded to ventilate the galleries more perfectly, and the patients are recreated, and return into the wards better disposed to rest.

The extremest difficulty is generally found in enforcing regular attention to the exercise of the patients employed in the workshops; but, if possible, all of them, including the tailors and shoemakers, always the most disinclined to move, should be induced to walk into the grounds for an hour every afternoon or evening.

It is not desirable to allow the patients who work on the

farm or in the gardens to be employed later than five o'clock. At that hour they should be collected, and conducted to their respective wards by the out-door attendants, whose duty it should then be to report anything particular in the conduct or the apparent health of those who are more under their observation than that of the ward-attendants. These patients have, of course, had sufficient exercise, and their greatest pleasure at this time is to sit down to tea, and then to read, or play at draughts, or cards, or bagatelle, or to rest and do nothing until supper-time. Many of them are disposed to be extremely regular in their attendance at the morning and evening prayers, and it is desirable that the hours of these religious services should be regulated with a view to their so being.

At five or at six o'clock the evening service should take place in the chapel; the patients being conducted thither as in the morning. After this service, a portion of the attendants, not exceeding one third, should be permitted to go out for the evening. Each attendant should have this permission twice in the week.

If the evening service is performed at five, the female patients should have their tea and bread and butter afterward. The male patients should sup at seven; the attendants being as careful as at dinner respecting the division and distribution of the bread, cheese, and beer allowed for this meal, and the conservation of order and good humour. This welcome meal usually disposes the men to go tranquilly to bed; and it is rather difficult to decide as to the preference to be given for a similar meal to the female patients instead of tea. To many of the women, however, the afternoon's tea is more satisfactory; and even some of the men would, I believe, prefer tea in the evening to their ordinary supper; and in some cases, the health of the patients requires this substitution.

After every meal, the attendants should be carefully accustomed to lock up all the knives, forks, spoons, dishes, &c., as

5

soon as they are made clean. The inconveniences arising from any neglect of this duty are innumerable.

Soon after seven, many of the patients like to go to their bedrooms, and to bed. The regular hour for doing so is eight—an hour doubtless felt by many to be much too early, particularly in summer time; but a later hour would be incompatible with the relief of the attendants, which, it may easily be supposed, is absolutely necessary to them after fourteen hours of activity during which they have scarcely sate down for a quarter of an hour at any one time, and have been from time to time agitated or excited, or had to contend with various difficulties, only to be estimated by those who occasionally devote even one hour to any one ward. In large asylums, these duties are also performed in an atmosphere which no ordinary system of ventilation can prevent from a deterioration productive of depressing effects. It becomes, therefore, indispensable to the effective performance of these duties day after day, that the attendants should have an opportunity of being at least one hour in the open air in the evening, before their supper hour, or before their own bedtime. By persuasion and proper management, the indisposition of some of the patients to go to bed so early as eight may generally be overcome. It is a general rule in some asylums, that the clothes of the patients should be taken out of their bedrooms at night, and wrapped up, and placed on the outside of the bedroom door. This is a necessary precaution as regards suicidal patients, who are disposed to tear their clothing, and convert it into the means of self-destruction. For the same reason they are sometimes only supplied with the ticking bed-clothing, in which blankets are sewed, and no sheets, or caps with strings, are allowed them. The same rule as respects the clothing must be observed when patients are violent, or dirty, or slovenly, or destructive, and in the habit of carrying knives, scissors, &c., about in the pockets of their dress. Such patients accumulate and hide under the bedding a variety of litter, which ought carefully to be removed. But there are a great many orderly, clean, and tranquil patients in an asylum, to whom these general rules are not found to be applicable; and as this leads first to its disuse in the rooms of such patients, and then to its neglect in other rooms where it is really required, the regulation ought to be understood to apply to certain cases only, and if acted upon generally in the cases of patients recently admitted, should in many instances be dispensed with after a short acquaintance with their habits. The same discretionary application of the regulations as to closing windows and window-shutters must, of necessity, be often intrusted to the attendants. As a general rule, every bedroom window should be shut at night in cold weather; but there are patients in whom the sense of heat is so distressing, that even in the coldest night they seem to require the admission of the external air into their bedrooms. The window-shutters should be carefully closed wherever there are patients disposed to injure the windows, or to make disturbing noises. In other cases, the patients who prefer not having the shutter closed, should be permitted to have it open; and some of them thus make a good use of the early light of the mornings in summer.

At this hour the attendant has to bethink himself of the appliances of dress, bedding, &c., required in the night, and which are then as much substitutes for restraint as those already mentioned as being to be thought of at ten a.m. for the day. Many patients are noisy or restless at night, who pass the days in tolerable tranquillity. One of the best preparatives for good sleep is exercise in the open air; and an evening walk may act as a sedative. Rest at night is also more likely to be enjoyed by those who have not been irritated in the day, or before going to bed, or sent to bed cold or hungry, or thirsty and feverish. A kind manner, a little bread, sometimes a supper of bread and cheese and porter, or ale; or arrow-root, with a little brandy; sometimes a glass of water, or a warm bath, may be better than any sedative in the materia medica. An attendant may soon learn the habits or peculiarities of his patients in those respects. Even a little tobacco or snuff will occasionally give a quiet night to a patient, who, without this indulgence, would be sleepless, or talk or swear for several hours.

There are patients who evidently suffer most when lying down ; there are some to whom the heat of a bed is intolerable. They have sensations of burning heat, scarcely known to the sane. These patients suffer for a length of time from the restlessness which every one knows who has ever known a bad night, but in a more intense degree. The old method of fastening down such patients in bed made them frantic ; and their cries proclaimed their excessive wretchedness. A dress suited to the weather ; a well-ventilated room ; cool drink; the application of cold water to the face and hands,—these are the remedies to which we instinctively resort when hot and sleepless ; and the attendants must be taught to administer them to those who are hot and restless from disorder of the brain and nerves.

One important part of an attendant's duty at locking-up time, is to ascertain that each patient is present in his bedroom, and then to lock every door. The galleries should afterward be kept free from unnecessary intrusion, and, with the exception of one moderate light in each gallery or passage, all the lights should be put out. When all this is done, the night attendants should enter on their duty, and all the rest be at immediate liberty.

It is difficult to make satisfactory arrangements for night-watching. If attendants sleep in any of the dormitories, they do not obtain sufficient rest, and no advantage arises from their discomfort as regards the numerous patients not in dormitories. If a certain number of the attendants take the night-duty in turn, they of course enter on this duty at the close of their ordinary duties, and more disposed to sleep than to watch. If the night-duty is divided into two watches, the number of attendants deprived of an entire night's rest is doubled, and general discontent is the result; which is a bad security for the efficient performance of any duty. If there are especial attendants for the night-watching alone, they can either have no employment in the day, or there is no more security for their watchful attention during the night than there is for the same vigilance in those who have been employed during the day. Yet the general watching of a large asylum during the night is of great consequence to many of the patients : some require food, cordials, medicine, cooling drink, or various medicines ; some become suddenly violent, and require timely attention, or become dangerous to others ; epileptic patients are constantly liable to severe attacks of their malady ; the paralytic, and those disposed to apoplectic seizures are subject to sudden and serious accidents ; and the suicidal require to be frequently visited. At Hanwell, two attendants sit up every night on the male side of the asylum, and two on the female side. They are allowed tea, coffee, butter, and sugar in addition to the ordinary rations of the day ; and they enter on their duty at eight o'clock in the evening. At that hour all the other attendants close the duties of the day by sending in their evening reports to the medical officers, stating the number of beds in their ward, the number of patients actually in the ward, the number of the absent, and also the seclusions, admissions, discharges, deaths, or other circumstances since they entered on that day's duties. They are then free from particular duties and responsibilities until the following morning at six. The first duty of the night-attendants is to examine the lists, left in the infirmaries, of those patients who require especial attention in the night. Each list should contain the name of the patient, the number of the ward, the number of the bedroom, and the number of the bed, in which the patient is. The list of things ordered for the night, should be immediately compared with the things actually provided, so that any deficiencies may be made up before the officers and other attendants have gone to bed. The best security for the proper performance of night duties, as of day duties, is such a government and treatment of the attendants as may engage their feelings on the side of their duty, and in the general management of the asylum.

At nine o'clock, the male and female attendants have supper in their respective halls; and care should be taken to make this a comfortable meal to them after the toil of the day. At ten o'clock, the attendants who have been out for the evening should return to the asylum—perhaps somewhat earlier in the winter; but no advantage arises from abridging their allotted time of relaxation in the fine evenings of summer, and the head attendant should prevent any irregularity which may cause them to go to bed supperless on their return. There is a great want of consideration in any rules which either exact their return at an unreasonably early hour, or omit all provision for their comfort when they do return. The attendants have often to visit friends who live far from the asylum, and who are too poor to entertain them: if, in addition to this, they are to return to a cheerless home, it is extremely unlikely that they will feel attached to it, or pursue their peculiar avocations in the asylum with the cheerfulness and good-will essential to their efficiency as the instruments of comfort or of cure to the patients. Their days and hours of leave should be days free, if possible, from anxiety; and every arrangement should be made that can ensure their entrance of the gate of the asylum, when they return, in a cheerful state of mind, refreshed by a short intermission of their duties, and fitter to go on with them. Every officer of common sense and common feeling must know how necessary all this is for himself; and it is most strange that it should be so often thought undeserving of attention as regards the attendants. The regulations of a prison can but produce in them the feelings of a turnkey, and such are not the feelings required in the attendants on the insane.

The great duty of the night-attendants is to visit the different wards several times in the night, and to administer the nourishment required by the weak and sinking, and the medicine ordered for the sick. Although their principal attention is generally required in the infirmaries, it should be faithfully extended to the wards in which the restless and refractory patients are placed, and not withheld from any part of the asylum. There is much inhumanity in any regulation debarring insane patients who are restless, or depressed, or sleepless, from the comfort of a little tea, because they are not in wards appropriated for the sick. Any resident officer who frequents the wards late at night will learn that there are many of the patients to whom a cup of tea, or of broth, or of sago, or sometimes a glass of water, or sometimes a few kind words, act as an immediate sedative, and contribute also to the great end of producing satisfaction in the day, as well as solace in the night. I have repeatedly witnessed the good effects of such attentions, and have known violent and noisy patients tranquillized for the night by being allowed water to wash their hands and face, and water to drink, and by having the bed made up afresh, and a cool dress put on, and a kind and cheerful good-night wished to them by kind-hearted attendants. To withhold all this, as if it were so much weak indulgence of the capricious, is to treat the insane as criminals, not as patients, and cannot be too strongly reprobated.

The officers of asylums who visit the wards after the patients are in bed, must show by their example how anxious they are to comfort the restless and to avoid disturbing those who are asleep. The attendants should wear cloth shoes, and the doors should be unlocked with the least possible noise. In addition to the light left in each gallery, each night-attendant should be provided with a lantern, and no candles should be taken into any bedroom except so protected. Patients who will not lie down should have cloth boots on, fastened by a small lock; and those who will only lie on the floor, should be placed in rooms of which the whole floor is a bed. I have lately been informed by Mr. Gaskell, so well known as the resident medical officer of the Lancaster Asylum, that the uncleanly habits of almost every patient in that large institution have been got the better of by means of the regular

visits of the night-attendants, who, it seems, have few or no
day duties in the asylum. If any accident or unusual circumstance takes place, the attendants should be able to ring a bell
communicating with the medical officer's bedroom.

In order to ensure watchfulness during the night, and to
give the attendants the means of proving it, I long since recommended the introduction of night-clocks into the asylum at
Hanwell. The dial-plate of these clocks turns round once in
twelve hours; and at each quarter of an hour, or half-hour, or
hour, the attendant is able to depress the one of the forty-
eight pegs which is exactly at the top of the dial-plate at that
time: but these clocks were immediately neglected. A physician to an asylum should have authority to enforce attention
to such matters, both in the attendants and officers. In a
small asylum he may himself see that all such duties are performed; but in a larger he requires help, and power to command it.

A little before six in the morning, the night-attendants call
up all the rest; they make out reports, in writing, of the state
of the wards, or of particular patients, during the night, and
of all especial occurrences; and then their duty ceases; and
they are not expected, at Hanwell, to take any share of the
ordinary ward duties of the day until after twelve o'clock.
Young, active, and healthy attendants do not suffer from the
recurrence of these night duties once in twelve or fourteen
nights; and, generally speaking, I have found them very
faithful in the performance of them.

Such are the ordinary daily and nightly duties of the attendants on the insane in an asylum. There are also some
duties which occur only on certain days in the week; and
there are many general attentions required, which are, in
reality, the whole mental or moral treatment of insanity
carried into practical effect. These, in their relations to the
patients, and to the qualifications and government of the attendants, and to the general constitution of an asylum, and the
character of its officers, still remain to be considered.

CHAPTER VI.

General Duties of Attendants in Asylums.—Their proper Government.—
Peculiar Duties of Attendants on Private Patients.

THERE are certain duties which require punctual performance, on the part of the attendants of a public asylum, at precise times, on certain days of the week only. Those of Sunday
will be particularly alluded to when ' I speak of the effect of
religious observances on the insane. On Monday morning,
the regular duties of the week begin by the attendants going
to the storeroom at seven, to receive the candles and soap,
and other articles required for the wards to which they re-
spectively belong, and also their own allowance of tea and
sugar for the week ; and at nine o'clock, they should take the
clothing requiring repair to the storerooms. The attendants
of the male wards should take such clothing to the general
storeroom ; and the female attendants should at the same, or
at some fixed hour, take to the female storeroom the needlework done in each ward in the previous week, and receive
from the female storekeeper a supply of work for the week
commencing. At a later hour, or about half-past nine, the
male and the female attendants should take their own clothes
to the laundry, where there should be a receiving room for this
purpose, having windows communicating with corridors from
both sides of the asylum. The frequent intermingling in the
laundry or kitchens of patients or attendants from both sides
of the asylum, leads to much loss of time, and, sometimes, to
greater inconveniences.

The various superintendents of work usually take the
charge of some new patients on a Monday; but in doing this,
and in receiving, on the female side, work to be done by the

5 §

patients during the week, they must not be accustomed to consider the asylum as a mere workhouse, in which the largest possible quantity of work is to be performed, nor as a prison, in which reluctance to work is a crime; but, on the contrary, be instructed to view the different employments as so many means of occupying the restless, diverting the thoughts of the melancholy, relieving the vacuity of the imbecile, turning morbid activity to useful account, and, in short, of contributing to the cure of all descriptions of patients. They should be encouraged to try to promote these good effects by their constant care of, and kindness to, the patients intrusted to them, and should receive expressions of just approval from the officers when those efforts have been in any degree successful.

Monday is at Hanwell one of the days on which new patients are received into the asylum. This important duty should not be wholly left to the attendants. The medical officer, and, in the case of female patients, the matron, or chief nurse, also, should have immediate notice of any new arrival. The patient should be received and welcomed kindly, and relieved from alarm or anxiety, by being assured that no unkindness will be experienced, and that being admitted to the asylum will lead to recovery, or to improved health and comfort. I am quite sure that a short conversation at this time produces lasting impressions; the patients feel that the removal is, in some way or other, an event of much importance to them, and their attention is, in such circumstances, directed, with more than usual acuteness, to whatever is said or done. They often afterward refer to any kind words then addressed to them.

When the officers have performed this duty, the new patient must be left for a time to the care of the attendants. Experienced male and female attendants are usually intrusted with the attentions then required. The patients are undressed; and if they have money, or trinkets, or a book, or little articles to which they attach some value, these should be taken care of for them. Very often, their chief possessions are pawnbrokers' duplicates, and these should be preserved. They always remember any losses to which they are subjected by carelessness as to these matters. Female patients are sometimes needlessly mortified by being deprived of their wedding-ring. All such things should be entered and described in a book, and numbered, and carefully kept, so as to be returned to the patient on recovery, or on amendment. The undressing of the patients should be done gently and kindly, and their own clothes, if not taken away by the parish officers, should be taken to the store-room, to be made clean, and kept for use, if in a state to be serviceable, when the patient is discharged. Each patient, on admission, should have a warm bath; and it must be remembered, that this luxury is so entirely new to most of the poorer patients as to be by no means welcome to them, although by some the comfort derived from it is gratefully acknowledged. During the undressing, and bathing, and drying, in all which operations the comfort of the patient should still be kept in mind, an opportunity is afforded for ascertaining the general condition of the patient, the state of the skin, the presence of bruises, &c., and the result of this observation should be reported to the medical officers. Too many unfortunate creatures are merely sent to county asylums to die; their emaciation, and ulcerations, and marks of restraints, are memorials of much past misery, and the kindest subsequent care is often extended to them in vain. They not unfrequently leave the workhouse or asylum from which they come, at such an hour as to lose their chance of dinner altogether; they are sometimes brought in open carts, in cold and wet weather, and their removal made unnecessarily miserable: the attendants should never permit them to remain long hungry and cold, and uncared for, after their arrival. When no proper care is omitted, it is often gratifying, after the patient has been an hour in the asylum, to see a poor, ragged, dirty, half-starved, sullen, wretched creature, transformed into a clean, decently-dressed, cheerful and hopeful person, disposed to be pleased

with everybody and everything : and this is a first step towards a cure.

Tuesday is, at Hanwell, one of the days on which the friends
and relatives of the patients are permitted to visit them. Much
discretion is required in the regulation of this indulgence.
Violent or excited patients should not be allowed to see their
friends soon after admission ; but those who are timid, and
melancholy, and attached to their relatives, should be allowed
to see them in the course of a week or a fortnight. Some
patients are invariably worse after interviews with their friends ;
and others grieve and pine if their relatives do not come near
them. Very frequent visits, or visits of long duration, are seldom or never attended with good effects. The attendants may
sometimes leave the patients and their friends together, but
not those of opposite sexes. In fine weather it gives the
patients much pleasure to walk about the grounds with their
friends ; and, under the general superintendence of the attendants, this ought to be allowed.

Rules should be put up at the gate, and in the visiting-
rooms, prohibiting any presents being brought to the patients
except tea, coffee, sugar, a little fruit, &c. ; and these rules
should be strictly enforced ; no other presents of any kind
being received without the sanction of the medical officers, and
the committee of the asylum. No attendant should be allowed
to take money, or other presents, from the friends of pauper
patients : poor as the friends are, they sometimes offer money,
out of their anxiety to ensure particular kindness to those
whom they visit.

Every male attendant on patients of the richer classes is expected to act in some measure as a valet ; and with pauper
patients, the attendant must be able to perform the functions
of barber, each male patient being shaved at least twice a
week, one of the days for this operation being Saturday. The
other day may be Wednesday, and this day and Sunday should
be the days for their having clean shirts. On a Thursday, the
clothes, linen, &c. of the female patients should be returned

by the superintendent of the laundry to the attendants of the different female wards; and on Friday, at nine o'clock, or some other convenient hour, the male attendants should go to the laundry, with patients selected to help in the duty, to fetch the clean clothes and linen of the male patients from the laundry to the wards.

On a Friday morning, also, every attendant in charge of a ward should give in a list, in writing, to the steward or storekeeper, of any household utensils or furniture required in the ward, or of any repairs necessary. In the evening of Friday, the female attendants should cause all the dirty clothes, &c. of each ward to be taken to the laundry. The male attendants should perform the same duty on Saturday. In some wards, a daily removal of clothes, &c. to the laundry, is, of course, required. As the cleanliness, comfort, and health of the patients is promoted by warm bathing, it should be a rule, that each patient, unless any particular reason makes it improper, should have a warm bath once a week; and Saturday is a convenient day for this attention. Where the patients are numerous, those of different wards should bathe on different days. Without vigilance on the part of the officers, this duty will often be neglected, or ill performed. The repaired clothing should also be given out from the storerooms, on Saturday, and provision should be made for dressing all the patients as neatly as possible on the Sunday morning, and particularly those who are anxious to make a respectable appearance at chapel. On the evening of Saturday, the attendants should see that none of the prayer-books, hymn-books, or bibles, allowed for the use of the wards, are missing; and when more are required, they should report the deficiency to the physician and chaplain.

Beside all these specified and particular duties, to be performed on stated days and at stated hours, there are general duties which devolve on the attendants, many of which scarcely admit of specific rules being laid down for them, but all of which should be performed in a general spirit of humanity.

An attendant must be expected to devote his whole time and
attention to the patients ; to consider himself the friend and
adviser of those who are separated from every other friend and
acquaintance, and the protector of those whom disorder of the
mind has incapacitated from taking care of themselves.   The
functions they are to perform are not merely those of servants;
they are the only sane persons always with the insane, and
their temper, their manners, their cheerfulness and activity,
their neatness and order, or the want of these qualities, will
exercise a continual influence on all who are committed to
their charge.   On very many occasions I have noticed the remarkable effects produced on a patient, and often on a whole
ward, by a change of attendant.   Dirty patients have become
cleanly, idle patients have become active, and morose patients
have become cheerful.   Contrary changes may not unfrequently be observed also, when the change is from a good
attendant to a bad one.

In asylums in which bodily restraints are never resorted to,
the great substitutes are continual superintendence and care.
From the hour of rising to the patient's bedtime, no ward
should, on any pretext whatever, be left without an attendant.
Without harassing the patients by useless and continual interference, the attendants must never be regardless of them, or
wholly unobservant of their conduct, their manners, their language ; and also of their dress, their appearance, their food,
their exercise, their occupations, or their amusements.   They
should always be ready to explain what a patient misunder-
stands, and to listen to and remedy little grievances which fret
the insane.   When the patients quarrel with one another, they
alone can prevent the beginning of strife, before blows are
struck ; and they will find that it is not difficult to do this, by
separating the disputants, and engaging their attention in
something else.   As regards the dress of the patients, their
care must often be relied upon for maintaining its cleanliness
and its decency, and every industrious attendant will find out
that there are many slovenly patients whose habits can be very

much improved. Some of them will doubtless try the patience of the attendants to the utmost, and require the same attentions many times a day; but this attention is part of the business of an attendant. By proper attention occasionally through the day, and the last thing at night, many patients may be relieved from the miseries consequent on a neglect of cleanly habits. Others may be encouraged to neatness and order. The attendant should consider it a duty to become acquainted with the characters of the patients under his care, and should be able to give a particular account of any of them when required: it is often important to the medical officers to be able to get information on which they can depend, relative to many circumstances of the patient's health and various propensities—as, whether they take food well or not, are active or indolent, good-tempered or morose, fond of work or of amusement, or of reading, or any particular occupation for which they require materials, or space, or other assistance; and the attendants have the most ample opportunities of knowing all these particulars. Some patients pass a large portion of their time in writing, or in making calculations on paper; and all their requests for writing paper, pens and ink, pencils, or books, should be complied with, of course within reasonable bounds. Their wishes on any subject should be made known to the physician;—as their wishes to be employed; any particular wish as to their clothing, or articles of furniture or decoration in their rooms; and especially any desire they may express to see the chaplain, or their minister; but no promises should ever be made to them which cannot be performed, and no deception of any kind ever be practised upon them.

Attendants should also be accustomed habitually to watch for the first signs of recovery, and to promote the progress that they see beginning. The indications of this, in an altered language, or dress, or manner, if neglected, may pass away for ever. Patients at this critical period require most delicate attention. Recollections, which were lost in the past excitement, come back irregularly, and with them, past feelings, as a remembered dream. Severe fits of sobbing and crying are then usual in female patients, and broken expressions relative to their past history, their errors, their griefs, their home, and those who loved them. They are, at this time, particularly sensible to kind words, but easily disturbed by violent impressions or painful emotions; and it is now, when an indiscreet word may retard recovery, that all the physician's trust, and all his hope, rest on the judicious aid of kind attendants.

These duties can only be reasonably expected from attendants of humanity and intelligence, who are treated kindly, governed justly and mercifully, and properly supported by the officers. If they look with dread to a passionate manner and words, which they expect to be manifested or addressed to them when the door of their ward is opened by an officer of the asylum, and are subjected to have degrading rebukes addressed to them, and threats, in the hearing of the patients, not only must their useful influence be lessened, but they must become disgusted with their duties, and sullen, and negligent, and too prone to direct some portion of their irritated feelings towards the patients, who have been already disturbed by the imperious tones and gestures of some officer, whose temper is unfitted to bear the unavoidable agitations and irritations of an asylum. The morning or evening visit of every officer should be the visit of a friend, alarming to none, unwelcome to none who endeavour to do their duty. It then becomes a highly useful means, of daily application, not always producing immediate results, but greatly influencing the character of the wards, and of the house, by daily repetition. These visits should be considered by the officers as the first and chief object of the day. If they are postponed until many other matters have been attended to, the officers run the risk of entering the wards with a discomposed temper, and consequently in a humour to discompose the attendants. Every inquiry should be made, and every order given, with calmness. Cruelty and neglect alone should be at once and openly reprimanded, yet not without some moderation. Deserving attendants will then cheerfully and truthfully communicate to the officers all that has passed in the ward, or all that they know; will represent any particular difficulties, sure of being aided in combating them; and will feel a gratification in pointing out any trifling change in any patient which indicates the first returning gleams of reason. Attendants who zealously endeavour to perform all their duties well should be treated with confidence, and allowed every reasonable indulgence. The natural pride they feel in the state of their ward, and in their influence over troublesome patients, should not be discouraged by frequent removals either of the patients or of themselves from one ward to another. Everything that affects them will be found to exercise a secondary influence on the patients; their health, their circumstances, their instruction, their mode of living in the asylum, their diet, the comfort of their sleeping-rooms, are all matters of much importance, generally attracting too little attention, and sometimes wholly overlooked in the arrangements of an asylum. Yet nothing can be more certain, than that attendants who lead an uncomfortable life are not likely to be in a state of mind to make patients comfortable. If it is forgotten that they have ordinary human feelings, or if they are treated as if presumed to be always dishonest and unworthy of trust, or are subjected to heartless or capricious refusals and mortifications when desirous of a little extra leave of absence, they cannot but lose all attachment to the officers, and all interest in the asylum. It is a mockery to tell attendants, who are not sure of their places for a day, that they are to devote themselves entirely to the patients, and to be themselves patterns of forbearance. Yet the want of devotedness on their parts is a want of that for which there is no substitute, and the want of forbearance in the attendants will lead to the worst consequences. So strictly connected is the proper government of an asylum with the welfare, and even with the safety of the patients. Unjust officers, or unjust rulers, make attendants indifferent or cruel, and indifferent or cruel attendants make the patients wretched.

When I had authority over the attendants at Hanwell, it was a rule with me never summarily to dismiss an attendant, except for cruelty; but never to overlook cruelty. There is no other security for the patients. Where a physician does not possess authority to do this, or any asylum is governed with slight regard to his general views, or other officers have authority quite independent of him, other faults will be punished by dismissal; but cruel conduct, the worst of all faults, will too often appear to be considered venial, and the attendants will too soon learn that common humanity may be disregarded, and the medical officers defied with impunity. The ignominious dismissal of an attendant on the insane is often a sentence of destitution; for unless they can meet with similar employment, they can seldom find any employment at all: it should therefore, on this account also, be reserved for cruelty or some serious offence alone; but for cruelty no excuse should be permitted. I should not dwell so much on this point of discipline if I did not believe it to be often incredibly undervalued, and with grievous effects on the patients.

It should be a rule that the attendants should never use violent or intemperate language; should never venture to strike or ill-treat a patient, or to employ the term punishment in relation to anything done to them. They should not even talk to the patients in a loud and scolding manner, nor give directions or collect the patients for dinner, or work, or exercise, or prayers with shouts and disturbance ; nor should they persevere in arguing with them, or contradicting them, or reproaching them for their faults. They should be always vigilant, should seldom interfere, but be ready for prompt interference when necessary. The general character of each ward should be tranquil, and yet the superintendence by eye and ear so perfect, that no person should pass through the ward, and no door be unlocked, without immediately attracting the attention, and occasioning the approach, of an attendant.

For protection in cases of great violence, the attendants must be intrusted with the power to seclude a patient; but the seclusion must always be immediately reported. The seclusion itself, which is merely putting the patient out of the gallery, or airing-court, into his bedroom, or into a padded room, and locking the door, should be effected without violence; and in cases of difficulty, by the united and prompt aid of many attendants, by whose conjoined exertions danger is best prevented, and the patient best overcome, without any doubtful, dangerous, and irritating contest between the patient and any one or two attendants. It may often be effected by persuasion alone, the patient having generally some consciousness of the desirableness of being quiet and alone. When the use of the strait-waistcoat and all other means of restraint was first forbidden at Hanwell, seclusion was resorted to for the protection of the attendants, and also because it best screened the patient from external excitement. It is now itself rarely resorted to, except as a remedial measure, and long seclusions have vanished with the wild confusion that prevailed when every excited patient was bound up in hard canvas and leather, or fastened in a coercion-chair.

The principle of promptly assisting one another should be rigidly adhered to by the attendants of an asylum. When the whistle, with which each attendant is provided, is blown, all within hearing should fly to the point from whence the signal proceeds, and every existing difficulty will then soon be overcome. The attendants are often averse to using this signal, and will encounter patients single-handed—a practice objectionable and dangerous, and which explains, without excusing, many injuries incurred both by patients and attendants. In such single contests somebody must be hurt. A strong array of attendants generally prevents resistance, and always makes it more safely as well as more easily overcome. But when a violent patient has been put into seclusion, or made to take a bath, or to dress or undress, by the united exertions of several attendants, attempts must afterward be made to conciliate him, and restore him to his self-esteem; and this will not be difficult when he has only yielded to numbers, who have merely overpowered him, or locked him up without hurting him.

Many patients being employed in assisting the attendants in their various ward duties, and also as helpers in the kitchens of the officers, it should be the general rule that all these patients should be treated with great kindness, but not spoiled by hurtful indulgences; otherwise, if employed in the wards, they appropriate to themselves more food and more beer than is good for them, and become tyrannical and insolent; and if employed out of the wards, their recovery does not proceed favorably. It thus happens that a quiet ward is sometimes disturbed by one very turbulent patient, who is too good a helper to be willingly parted with by the attendants. Those who are employed in the kitchens of the officers will enjoy, by this change of place, all the advantage of removal to a convalescent house, if the servants of the officers are capable of taking proper care of them. The house-servants should always conduct them from the wards in the morning, and back to the wards at night; should be considered responsible for their safety, and for their neatness and general good conduct, and should take them to chapel with them. No patients, however, should be employed in this manner without the knowledge and sanction of the medical officers. I have known surprising recoveries take place in patients employed in the matron's kitchen, and many very gratifying ones in the general kitchen, and in the houses of the officers; but I have also not unfrequently known recovery interrupted by the employment of patients in such situations, under irritable or incompetent servants, who were left in ignorance of the general rules and principles of the asylum.

Visitors to an asylum are generally anxious to derive information from the attendants; and when the attendants are ignorant, or ill-affected to the asylum, many wrong impressions are thus produced. The attendants also sometimes obtain money from visitors, and sometimes from the friends of the patients, or receive perquisites from the patients themselves, or sell things to them. All this should be strictly guarded against. Against the latter objectionable practices, the best preservative is identical with the best security for the proper performance of all their duties, namely, the selection of respectable attendants, giving them a liberal remuneration, increasing with length of service, and making their situation so generally comfortable, as to induce them to wish to retain it.

The whole life of the numerous incurable patients in county asylums must take its character from the attendants, and be agitated or tranquil, passed in misery or in content, according to the qualifications possessed by those in whose sole and immediate charge and power they must necessarily be for the greatest part of every day. Everything that a judicious committee wishes to be carried into effect,—every comfort that the benevolence of the officers would wish to confer,—every appliance of daily treatment,—every curative means, will be either realized or withheld, according to the character of the attendants. They are the instruments by which every great and good intention is brought into hourly practice. It is not necessary to say more, to prove how important it is that they should be well chosen, well governed, well taken care of, well supported in their duty, and well paid.

Patients of a richer class than those usually found in a county asylum are yet as much dependent for care during the severity of their attack, kindness during the progress of the malady, and delicate attention when convalescence begins, as the poorest lunatic in the world. The attendants on such cases are usually well remunerated, and appear to lead an easy, if not an idle life; but their situation is really irksome and anxious, and they do not always enjoy so many intervals

of relaxation as the attendants in a county asylum.   It seems
often to be most unreasonably expected, that an attendant on
a private patient should be never absent from the patient,
night or day, for months together.   The smallest leave of
absence is assented to with reluctance.   This extreme want of
consideration must have the effect of incapacitating the attendants for the proper and cheerful performance of the
peculiar duties required.   Their respectability and their so-
briety are points of great consequence, for they are often
intrusted with the general management of single patients ;
but to expect them to lead a life of entire monotony, with an
abnegation of every form of mental relief, is entirely opposed
to their usefulness as mental instruments.   In this respect the
regulations of asylums, and the customs of private families, of
which one member is insane, usually indicate equal ignorance
of the commonest principles of proper treatment.   Although,
therefore, it is a matter of great regret, it cannot excite surprise, that so few persons of education, of either sex, are to be
found ready to apply their services to the insane, either as
attendants or companions.   The richer patients, who are
either in separate residences, with attendants, or in asylums
in which patients of no other class are taken, are indignant,
in their worst state, on finding themselves under the control
of persons who are not superior in manners or education to
their own servants; and they suffer still more, when convalescent, from the want of conversation suited to them.   When
the terrible infliction of insanity falls upon the rich, it finds
them more prepared to exhibit all its most varied and agitated
aspects, and perhaps less open to consolation from sympathy
or kind attentions, than the poor.   Their intellectual faculties
are more developed than those of the class living by manual
labour, and their affections are less open to simple impressions.
These circumstances render some parts of the moral treatment
easier, but some also more difficult, than they are found to be
in the case of the pauper lunatic.   The mental appliances, and
resources capable of remedial adaptation to them, are more

numerous : but their long-indulged passions and propensities frequently resist the treatment which appeals to the sympathies or affections; and attentions, which would soothe and charm those little accustomed to kindness, are regarded by them as merely matters of right. Thus it often happens that they are incurably imperious, or suspicious, or disobedient; less grateful for laborious services, and less easily attached; a long course of consistent kindness will often fail to conciliate them, which is seldom the case with patients of humbler condition. They are also more capricious, and more ingeniously mischievous, as well as more imaginative and fanciful, and more apt to be involved in deep and intricate delusions. All this makes the care of them by ordinary attendants very difficult, and very trying to attendants of the highest qualifications.

I have taken pains to ascertain the real feelings of patients of the higher classes on these subjects, and I know that although they may be conscious that their own conduct is often inconceivably provoking, the negligence of their attendants, or any assumption of entire authority over them by uneducated persons, is intolerable to them; and they complain of suffering from various acts of petty tyranny, when the attendants are of an unkind disposition, which they conceal from the superintendent of the house, out of fear of irritating the attendants further, and of causing them to make representations which may lessen the chance of their liberation. The proprietors of private houses cannot be too anxious to investigate every complaint made by the patients; the complaints will sometimes be groundless, but, on the other hand, much petty cruelty may be long concealed.

Every part of the management of the insane requires to be modified according to the previous habits of the patients. I generally observe, that the best educated of those whom we receive at Hanwell appear at first to be content, but soon become restless and dissatisfied. They have usually been subjected to rudeness before admission, perhaps have been put into a

station-house for a night, or, more commonly, have been placed
in a workhouse, and unceremoniously addressed, or roughly
questioned, by persons in parochial or magisterial authority,
and have felt the various miseries of friendless destitution. On
arriving at the asylum, its ordinary comforts are found to be
strongly contrasted with what they have lately been exposed
to, and produce an immediate satisfaction. The mere novelty
of the scene interests their cultivated observation, and they
feel a kind of pride in submitting to the regulations of the
place. But after a month or two the monotony of even so
cheerful an asylum as Hanwell wearies them. They lan-
guish for want of more numerous and more varied impressions, and suffer nearly as much as they always seem to
do in private asylums, from the difficulty of satisfying the
peculiar requirements of their minds. That patients of such
habits must be extremely difficult to manage singly, separated
from their families, and unoccupied in any of their usual pur-
suits, will readily be conceived ; and their comfortable management demands a fertility of resources rarely to be met with in
an attendant. At the same time such patients require all the
ordinary attentions of the insane ; care as to their dress, their
food, their general health, their exercise and rest, their habits,
manners, and language ; being often singularly troublesome in
all these particulars ; and, perhaps, taking a morbid delight
in troubling and teasing those who wait upon them ; demanding almost incessant attentions, and repaying all by abuse.
Against all this, and much more, the attendants on gentlemen
and ladies have to struggle, and all the time to endeavour to
preserve in their patients some remnants of their former
habits, and to restore all those conventionalities of rank which
insanity seldom respects.

There are, however, some peculiarities of mental character
in the insane of the educated classes, which may encourage
and will reward the watchful care of an attendant. In persons of cultivated intellect, over whom insanity is impending,
or on whom it has fallen, the resistance to the dominion of

morbid impulses is usually longer and more successfully kept up than among the ignorant and uneducated; and more readily resumed as soon as convalescence begins to dawn. Their self-control may therefore be expected to be more easily excited as a remedial means; they are more sensible to well-timed reproof, and of the honour of contending with a malady which has well-nigh mastered them for ever. The extremely delicate task of attempting to take advantage of these characteristics must often devolve on the attendant alone; and it demands all the qualifications which I have now so often referred to. It can, indeed, scarcely in fairness be left wholly in their hands; for the utmost judgment is required in trying to accomplish it, and in determining how far to proceed in attempts to renew the exercise of the mental faculties, and when to desist from persuasions and to abstain from arguments.

CHAPTER VII.

*Concluding Chapter. — Religious Services in an Asylum. — Schools.—
Government of Asylums.—Treatment of Officers.—Position and Duties
of the Medical Superintendent.*

THE abolition of the old methods of coercion, and the consequent mitigation of the symptoms of insanity, have led, as a
natural and happy consequence, to the recognition of the pos-
session, by insane persons, of many of the feelings which relieve their affliction from debasement, as well as of surviving
intellectual faculties, capable of cultivation. To the preservation of these feelings, and to the resuscitation of these
faculties, after various approaches to moral torpor and death,
a more enlightened treatment has now extended itself. Attempts which would have been vain in connexion with the old
and shocking system of dungeons and blows, have become
reasonable, and promise to become more and more successful,
under a milder government, more consonant to civilized and
Christian communities. Thus, into places of abode where
words of kindness were once never heard, ministers of a religion of mercy have penetrated, and to those to whom tones
of reproach or violent menace were once alone familiar,
spiritual consolation has been successfully addressed, and
lessons of instruction have been afforded with advantage.
This is part of the superstructure for which the abolition of
restraints was but a foundation. Having removed from disordered minds every removable source of pain, vexation, or
fear, it now remains to be seen what further can be done;
how much may yet be preserved; what can yet be restored of
the faculties, the loss of which deprives human life of its best

privileges, and throws the unhappy afflicted person out of his proper rank in the creation.

The institution of religious services in asylums has created new and peculiar duties for the officers; and although I can readily conceive the apprehension with which the medical superintendents of some asylums regard this subject, and know how unjust it generally would be to ascribe such apprehensions to indifference, I am quite satisfied, that with reasonable caution in the exercise of his peculiar duties, a chaplain may become a valuable officer in asylums for the insane.   It is unfortunately true, that no cause of mania, melancholia, and imbecility is more common than a gloomy religion, which excludes the idea of God's mercy so carefully, and brings forward God's judgments so prominently, as to alarm, and depress, and enfeeble many enthusiastic and weak persons who are exposed to its doctrines.   Among persons of education, and particularly among women, I believe that nearly one half of the cases of derangement of mind arise from this perversion of religion alone.   Exciting meetings, enthusiastic exhortations, false reports of wild missions, foolish biographies of sickly and delirious children, incoherent tracts, and books of unfruitful controversy, constitute all the intellectual exercises of these sincere and misguided persons. All elegant literature, and almost all science, is kept from them, as demoralizing or tending to unbelief.   All cheerful avenues of thought are forbidden to them.   A restless, meddling, dictatorial spirit, much opposed to real charity, assumes the guise and name of benevolence and religious zeal.   By degrees, the mind—so ill-exercised, so ill-governed, so excited—becomes weakened, and then the mask falls to the ground.   Spiritual and worldly pride, idle prophesyings, convictions of eternal wrath, fierce denunciations of neighbours, or parents, or children, or relatives, and, too often, despair and attempts at self-destruction, declare that madness has supervened.   Knowing all this, by daily observation, I feel as strongly as any physician can do, the danger of misapplying religious attentions; but I still

believe that many insane persons are capable of deriving much
satisfaction from being permitted to attend the services of
their church: and that a good and prudent clergyman may
become a useful auxiliary to a physician, by correcting fana-
tical delusions, moderating spiritual conceit, vindicating God
from the unjust views of his creatures, and reviving every hope
that is permitted to the imperfect and the penitent. Of course
it is only in the character of a physician to the insane that I
presume to speak of this serious subject at all.

There can be no doubt in anybody's mind, that the arrangements made in an asylum for the observance of Sunday may
be such as to assist the general plan of a physician whose endeavours are understood to be directed to curing his patients
by tranquillizing the excited brain, and soliciting such faculties
as are disordered or oppressed to ancient and customary exercise. Many of the patients keep exact account of seasons,
and months, and weeks, and days. Their recollections of
Sunday, as a day of rest from toil, or a day of mental repose,
and quiet and cleanliness, in every rank except the most abject, are not effaced; and the customs of an asylum should
accord with them. On Sunday morning the attendants should
see that every patient capable of being dressed neatly, should
be supplied with all the means of being so. They should take
care that every patient desirous of going to the chapel should
be ready to go when the bell rings; and they should remind
some, who take little notice of these preparations, that if they
wish it they can also attend. All who can read, and can take
care of books, should be supplied with prayer-books and
hymn-books. A certain proportion of the attendants, themselves in Sunday dress, should accompany the patients to
chapel, preventing their entering with indecorous haste, or
crowding on the same benches, or dispossessing those well
known to have some favorite seat. There are some patients
whose peculiarities make it desirable to place them immediately under the observation of the attendants; and the
epileptic should be induced, if possible, to sit on the lowest

benches, so as easily to be removed if a paroxysm comes on. During the service, if any patient is observed to be becoming fidgetty, an attendant should go and sit by the patient's side; or, if necessary, walk quietly out of the chapel with him. To know when *not* to interfere is a valuable knowledge in an attendant: several patients have odd and restless habits, and yet, after getting up once or twice, will sit down and be tranquil through the rest of the service. If a patient has a fit, he should be at once removed, with as little noise as possible, by three or four attendants. These attentions should be systematically given; and when such is the case, such events produce no disturbance in an insane congregation.

Those who have never before been in the chapel of an asylum for the insane are generally surprised to find that the patients join in the responses and singing, in a manner which some sane congregations would do well to imitate. The attendants should be trained to assist the patients, and set them an example in these respects, uttering the responses with moderate voices, and also singing, if able to sing. For this reason, as well as others, I should wish to have the attendants instructed in singing.

If the officers desire that the attendants and patients should conduct themselves satisfactorily in all these respects, they must themselves set the example. They should not come into the chapel without prayer-books and hymn-books, as if they dropped in by accident, or were merely there to watch the patients. If friends accompany them, they should interdict loud talking as they approach the chapel door, and any injudicious manifestation of excited curiosity. The officers, their families, and their servants should be punctual and constant in their attendance, and as careful in their demeanour as if they were in the parish church. The services should begin with great exactness, and never exceed one hour. At Hanwell, the organ is now played by a convalescent patient: it was formerly played either by female officers or members of the officers' families. I should, however, prefer engaging a regular organist for this duty, in order to its steady and consistent performance, any interruption or uncertainty of which confuses the patients.

It would scarcely be proper for me to say anything of the chaplain's duties in the chapel, except that they should always commence with exactness, and that some passages in the Scriptures, and some kinds of sermons, being peculiarly likely to be misapplied, or to produce useless or unsalutary terror, must be abstained from in reading and preaching. I have known great faults committed by a disdainful disregard of this precaution; and I have no hesitation in saying that it would be better to have no clergyman at all in an asylum than one who should unfortunately think it beneath the dignity of his office to pay attention to it. In some of the several Annual Reports which I have published, I have endeavoured to express my sense of the kind and able assistance derived from the Rev. J. T. Burt, the former chaplain, to whom we were also indebted for the formation of the asylum-schools. I have now much pleasure in bearing my testimony to the kindness and judgment of his successor, the Rev. J. May. When the physician has perfect confidence in the chaplain, many of the restrictions generally laid on that officer may be relaxed, and a free intercourse allowed with the patients; always, however, with a general reference to the physician's principles of treatment, and, in special cases, with especial reference to his opinion and wishes.

My Reports have also recorded my observations on the effects of the chaplain's office on the patients; I can but briefly repeat them. One of the effects is the exercise, in many patients, of a temporary control over themselves. I disapprove of taking noisy and ill-behaved patients to chapel, because I wish that a habit of tranquillity should be created and invariably preserved there; but sometimes a patient who has formerly been noisy, and who is still rather excited, will so earnestly petition to be allowed to go to chapel again, and make such solemn promises to keep quiet, that the trial may be made, and it will generally prove successful. There are many patients at Han-well who attend the chapel every day in the year, or every Sunday, and sit in the same place; and the decorous gravity of their demeanour would little prepare the observer for the general incoherence of their thoughts and discourse. After the service, the patients walk through the galleries to their respective wards with as much order as a village congregation. I have witnessed the same order both during and after the service in the asylum of the Salpêtrière, in Paris; several of the patients being taken to the parish church within that great establishment every Sunday, and having a sermon preached to them afterward in the school-room.*

The patients who do not belong to the Church of England should, of course, be permitted to see their minister. Except the Irish Catholics, however, I have scarcely ever found a patient, not of the English Church, desirous of seeing a minis-ter or priest. The Roman Catholics appear, generally, to derive more consolation from religious reading, and to be more easily cheered in their spiritual views, than the patients of our own church; and religious despondency seems to be rare among them.

It is not necessary to say more on this subject. The zeal of a good clergyman will be the best security for his more especial attentions to the sick who cannot be taken into the chapel; and if his duties are to be efficiently performed, con-fidence must be reposed in him. There are, however, kinds of exhortation, and descriptions of books and tracts, so mis-chievous, that the physician should have power to protect his patients from their influence: the latter are the real poison of religious literature, and have, I sincerely believe, driven many scrupulous minds to insanity. All books should be submitted to the physician's inspection before being circulated among the patients; and there should be frequent communication between the chaplain and physician concerning the nature and

* See Appendix.

effects of any particular conversations held with the patients. As some of the patients are anxious, occasionally, to receive the sacrament, it should be required of the attendants of each ward to make out lists of all such as desire to communicate, at such times as the chaplain may appoint; the lists should be submitted to the physician, and lastly, to the chaplain; so that, either for medical or other reasons, none should be admitted whom the ceremony might disturb, or who might in any way interrupt its solemnity.

I believe the experience of all the chaplains of asylums has taught them, that there is great difficulty in ascertaining to what extent their most anxious endeavours are really serviceable, and that all their attempts should be characterized by moderation. It is, indeed, not only of consequence that the clergyman, but that every one who converses with the insane, should exercise a sober discretion, and preserve an even and unexciting tone. An injudicious topic, or the use of an unguarded expression, will sometimes renew the cerebral irritation, and retard recovery. The religious fervour which springs from mere physical excitement must not be incautiously encouraged. The tears and self-accusations of mental despondency must not be regarded as a wholesome and welcome penitence. These are among the irregular phenomena of convalescence; and such errors of interpretation will be fatal to recovery.

Again, and for the last time in the course of these pages, I must observe, that neither can religious services have their due effect, nor tranquil feelings exist in an asylum, without frequent and severe interruption, if mechanical restraints are permitted, or any habitual tyranny is exercised. Patients subject to endure or witness the imposition of restraints, or exposed to habitual neglect, regard those who have the care of them as enemies, gaolers, and tyrants; suspect their piety, and reject and despise their inconsistent attempts to reconcile them to misery. The whole system of an asylum must be consistently humane, or it will not be effectual.

Independently of religious instruction, attempts have been made, with success, in many asylums in Great Britain and Ireland, on the Continent, and in America, to improve the general education and exercise the imperfect faculties of several of the patients contained in asylums, and to instruct others in reading, writing, arithmetic, geography, drawing, singing, &c. The abuse of what is called education, and a morbid anxiety for mere intellectual acquirement, are as prevalent in society as is an abuse of religion; but no just argument can thence be drawn against attempts to restore the faculties of the mind to moderate activity. Such attempts only require the same discretion as attempts to teach religious truths to the insane, or even as attempts to induce them to occupy themselves in work. At Hanwell, the experiment began under the superintendence of the Rev. Mr. Burt, in 1842, by the establishment of reading-classes. The number of patients in each class varied from six to fourteen; each patient read a few passages in turn, and illustrative pictures, maps, and observations were employed. As the lessons proceeded, it was found that more command was obtained by the patients over their powers of attention, and that they read with more confidence. Some who had lost the habit of reading reacquired it; some who had forgotten the art of writing learned to write again; and some learned to write who had never known how to hold a pen. Their copy-books furnish gratifying evidence of the progress of the writers. In the first page of some of them you find nothing but unmeaning marks or idle scrawling; the next page shows more attention; the next is an imperfect but careful copy; and there is a gradual amendment afterward. Attendance at the schools was a source of evident pleasure, and it was so arranged as scarcely to interfere with any of the ordinary employments of the asylum, and, consequently, was scarcely extended to the most intelligent of the patients; so that the difficulties to be met by the schoolmaster and schoolmistress were very great. There were also no separate rooms for the schools. But with these and

6 §

other disadvantages, the spectacle afforded by the schools was
to me, and I believe to almost every officer of the asylum,
most gratifying: instruction had been, to a greater or less
extent, afforded to about 80 female and 120 male patients;
and it was with the deepest concern that I at length unex-
pectedly found the schools closed, by order of the visiting
justices.

It is mortifying to have to mention what seems like an
acknowledgment of the failure of this plan; but I have un-
diminished confidence in the judgment and kindness of the
magistrates, when they are not studiously deceived; and still
entertain no doubt that the schools will be re-established at
Hanwell. For proofs of the practicability of such an attempt,
and of the results that may be expected, I would refer to the
official Report of the Inspectors-General on the Irish Asylums
for 1844; and especially to the Report on the Armagh Asylum;
to Dr. Brigham's Reports of the State Lunatic Asylum at
Utica, U. S., for 1844, 1845, and 1846; to the actual state
of the schools in the great French asylums, and especially at
the Bicêtre, of which a notice will be found in the Appendix;
to an interesting work of M. Seguin, 'On the Moral Treatment
of Idiots,' (1846), of which a translation is preparing by
Dr. Forbes Winslow; and to M. Voisin's treatise; to the latest
Reports of the Lancaster Asylum; and to the 'Observations' of
Dr. De Vitré, the physician to that asylum, 'on the necessity
of an extended legislative protection to persons of unsound
mind;' and, lastly, to the interesting facts recorded in the
section 'Mental Exercise,' in Dr. Browne's Seventh Annual
Report of the Crichton Institution at Dumfries, (1846.)

I have still to make a few remarks on the *government* of
asylums; a subject closely connected with the well-doing and
the recovery of the patients; and although I feel the difficulty
of avoiding the influence of some personal recollections or
impressions, I still more strongly feel that I am recording
opinions which will be read not only where all such personal

associations and impressions are unknown, but when all who were concerned in them will be forgotten.

An asylum ought to be neither a prison nor a workhouse; but a place of refuge and of recovery from all the mental distractions incidental to mankind.   Comfort in all cases, and recovery in many, are the attainable results of proper agencies directed to the remains of affection and intelligence existing in every case, and varying in all cases.   The object, therefore, of every law and regulation of an asylum, and of its whole constitution, should be to bring to bear on all the patients such an amount of intelligence and benevolence as may soothe many, and direct all, and raise each patient to the point of cure attainable in each particular case.   All the details should be part of one harmonious whole.   The patients should be accustomed to look on the attendants as their constant friends and guardians; the attendants should expect the visits of the officers with pleasure, and rely upon them for advice and encouragement; the officers should be animated by the example of a humane and intelligent medical superintendent; and he and they should look forward to the occasional visits of the directors with confidence.   If the patients fear the attendants, and the attendants dread the officers, and the officers look forward to committee days as days of insult, all must go wrong.

There is so much that is peculiar in the management of an asylum, that the wonder is, not that such institutions should often be mismanaged, but that governing bodies, not one member of which can be supposed to have had opportunities of acquiring much previous knowledge of the subject, should, upon the whole, acquit themselves of this duty so creditably. The true requirements of a member of such body comprehend not only an attention to finance, and a strict enforcement of regulations, but a consideration of the human character, and of everything that can affect the feelings, and stimulate or depress the exertions, of those officers to whom the direction of infirm minds is intrusted.   It must sometimes happen that these requirements are wanting; and when that is the case, the governing body, without courage to leave proper authority in the hands of the superintendent, interfering in turn with every officer, and distrustful of all, without reliance even on attendants chosen by themselves, will change their regulations frequently, making the bonds of discipline tighter, now here, now there, until they are irksome to all, and really useful to none. The laws of the asylum in one month will not be the laws of the asylum the next month; depending sometimes on mere temporary expediency, sometimes on motives merely personal, and very seldom on any general principles. Causes of this kind cannot but be supposed at least to be connected with the very frequent changes occurring among the officers of the principal asylums of England. No officer understands his position, or is sure of it; and the patients are seldom permitted long to enjoy the benefit of any one consistent system.

The direction of an asylum ought to be such as to create a very different spirit. It should be such as to declare, in every act, a remedial intention ever present to the directors. It should be calm, uniform, and just, dictated by a warm philanthropy, and should inspire confidence throughout all the ramifications of the internal administration; so that all the duties of all the officers, and attendants, and servants, from the highest to the lowest, should be performed cheerfully, and in an enlightened, benevolent, and uniform spirit, concentrating all its good influences on the patients, for whom the public has provided asylums, and to benefit whom the officers and servants are appointed and paid. All the rules and regulations of the asylum should breathe the same spirit, and then no excuse would exist, and none should be admitted, for disregarding them; and these rules should seldom be changed, and never without long notice, and great consideration.

These are principles which cannot be departed from without producing great uneasiness and discomfort in asylums, and without adding to the afflictions of the insane, and rendering the efforts of the superintendent or director a perpetual and painful struggle against influences opposed to all his remedial indications. I believe, also, that these are principles which can only be carried into effect in any asylum by the selection of a medical director, in whom the governing body or committee reposes full confidence, and to whom it imparts full authority over every other officer, and over every attendant and servant in the house. So trusted, and so armed, supposing that common prudence has been consulted in his appointment, every motive that can act upon an intelligent, honorable, and benevolent mind will induce him to consider the task he has undertaken, to mature his plan, and to ensure its success by means of officers in whom he can trust, and attendants on whose fidelity he can rely. The whole character of an asylum, in such cases, must be so conspicuously good or bad, that the directors can never be long exposed to any painful doubts on the subject. If it is good, the less they interfere the better. Observing everything, superintending everything, having everything explained to them, they should refrain from active interference; confine themselves chiefly to suggestions; as much as possible abstain from details; and wholly and entirely withhold from meddling with points of discipline in the wards. If the character of the asylum becomes bad, it must, with such a constitution, become soon and visibly bad altogether; and they have their remedy, and should apply it. It is not reasonable to say that this is difficult; for it is well known that the officers of such institutions can very easily be got rid of, even for reasons less important.

Seven years of close observation of the management of Hanwell have convinced me that no mistake can be more unfortunate than that of placing the direct government of an asylum for the insane in any other hands than that of a physician. Any other governor will find that he can only avoid being mischievous by avoiding all kind of interference. He must be idle, or he can scarcely be harmless. If he supports the physician, such support should not be required; if he opposes him, or controls him, the welfare of the patients is sacrificed, and the asylum is ruined.   To put a gallant officer in such a position, or to transfer a governor to an asylum from a prison, is to place such individuals in a position in which all their previous experience becomes nearly useless, and for which nearly all their acquired habits disqualify them. To intrust such officers with the choice of attendants on the patients, the regulation of their duties, and even with the classification of the patients, can only lead, by a succession of mistakes of lamentable consequence, to utter confusion.   It will readily be conceded that the regulations of a camp or a garrison can have little in them applicable to an asylum; but it will not, perhaps, so easily be granted that everything, and the manner of everything, that is considered suitable to a prison, is inappropriate and wrong as applied to an asylum for the insane.   It may be difficult for a magistrate to believe this, but nothing is more certain.

Without much forbearance and discretion, a visiting physician, non-resident, may become as mischievous as a non-medical governor.   Very few of the observations which I have to make on the influence of a medical superintendent have reference to a physician who is, by the nature of his office, reduced to the situation of a mere visitor, and cannot acquire the intimacy with the patients, or have that authority, or rather that paternal influence over them which is required to enable him to do much good.   The effects produced by his visits must be, as his visits are, occasional; and the perpetual influence requisite to produce great, general, and constant results must rest with those officers who live entirely in the asylum; and with whom a visiting physician can seldom interfere without doing harm.   Upon them alone devolves the important daily duty of visiting all the patients, and not only of prescribing for real, and sometimes for imaginary bodily ailments, but of examining the daily state of the refractory or the secluded; of directing the temperature and warmth of the wards, and of maintaining an orderly attention to all the regulations of the asylum : they alone have also the daily opportunities necessary for the prompt hearing and remedying of grievances, and healing of differences ; and their frequent visits, if so regulated as to leave each ward more comfortable than they find it, are the great remedies for which a visiting physician has very inferior opportunities.

In asylums which do not contain more than 400 patients, the medical superintendent chiefly requires an assistant to make up the medicines ; and there is, indeed, no such assistant in many asylums of that size. In a larger asylum, more assistance becomes necessary, and the assistants should either be appointed by the physician, or should act under his direction, communicating with and reporting to him on all subjects, and not making direct communications or suggestions to the committee. The duty of seeing every patient twice, or even once a day, prescribing for those who are sick, listening to the representations and complaints of others, giving directions for the special attentions required in particular cases, ascertaining that nothing important is omitted in the diet, clothing, exercise, classification, and general management of all the patients, examining new patients, keeping records and registers of cases, and attending to all the applications incidental to his office, becomes extremely laborious for one medical officer, when the patients exceed 300 in number, and impossible when the number exceeds 400. But the medical assistants should be expected in all things to conform to the plans of the physician, and he should have authority to direct them in their duties, and the times of performing them, and to require their co-operation, not only in the general duties of a superintendent of an asylum, but in any inquiries and investigations for which a large asylum affords opportunities. They should be required to keep journals of the cases, and diaries of the particular occurrences of each day ; but these diaries or daily reports should be made to the physician, and not to the committee, except where the physician is not a resident

of the asylum.   The attendants should make evening reports
to the assistant medical officers and the matron : the assistants
and the matron should report to the physician; and the
physician alone to the committee.

The matron of an asylum is usually chosen by the governing
body ; but it is a great evil in an asylum when this officer is
made of too much importance, and led to consider herself
independent of the physician, and has the power—by sending
away the attendants on his female patients, choosing others
without reference to him, and moving them from ward to
ward—to interfere in the most direct and mischievous manner
with highly important parts of his treatment.   A matron to
an asylum may be a valuable auxiliary to the medical officers,
and the means of doing much good ; of which I have had
some personal experience.   But matrons are generally spoiled
as auxiliaries to the medical officers, by a pardonable leaning
to female influence on the part of all committees, who are
pleased with the studious deference apparently paid to their
opinion, and really paid to their power; and thus the matron
becomes the only companion of the governors through the
wards, and almost the only source of their information ; and
it is the consequent fault of matrons of many institutions to
usurp authority, and to endeavour to exclude the medical
officers from all interference with the female side of the house,
beyond that of prescribing drugs.   Their influence, also, with
the governing bodies is not always exerted in the direction of
humanity or kindness, and their government of the nurses is
too often unjust and unfeeling.   I am very sorry to say it,
but in the generality of examinations made, or inquests held,
in hospitals or workhouses, or asylums, the matrons do not
appear to advantage, and are too often found to be the most
effective agents for harsh purposes.   There is reason to believe,
also, that in some asylums in which mechanical restraints are
yet employed, their abolition has been prevented by the
influence of the matron.   A woman's influence in an asylum
ought to be of a very different kind; and it is but just

to say, that in some remarkable, though too rare instances, such it has been. Upon the whole, however, I believe that where the matron of an asylum is not the wife of the superintendent, it would generally be productive of harmony to have no matron, but in her stead, a head nurse and an assistant nurse in each ward, superintendents in the different workrooms, the storeroom, and laundry; and, perhaps, a chief nurse over all, whose duty it should be to carry the superintendent's plans into effect on the female side of the house, reporting to him alone all circumstances appearing to call for his attention. The government of the female side of an asylum would then be assimilated to that of the male side, where, certainly, more order generally prevails, fewer complaints are made by the patients, fewer changes take place in the attendants, and fewer disagreements among the officers. This arrangement prevails in France, and in some of the asylums in the United States.

The medical superintendent of an asylum should have nothing to do with the steward's department, the supervision of which should rest with the committee. The steward's duty should be, to provide everything that the physician represents to the committee as necessary for the patients, and, together with the housekeeper, to exercise a general control over all domestic matters, including what may be termed the domestic habits of the attendants; but neither of these officers should interfere with the management of any patients except those employed by them.

Supposing all the officers of an asylum to be well selected, and a proper degree of authority vested in the medical superintendent, it seems desirable that the committee or governing body should place such a degree of confidence in them, as to exclude from the regulations all minute restrictions from which no good effects can ensue to the patients. In this respect, prison discipline at present taints the constitution of asylums; and medical and other officers, who have undertaken the peculiar task of regulating the mental as well as the bodily health of the insane, are needlessly harassed by rules and observances which interfere with their private life and domestic freedom. The medical superintendent should have power, within reasonable limits, to grant leave of absence to the officers and attendants. They sometimes require it on emergencies which prevent their waiting for the decision of a committee ; and the chief medical officer ought to be a competent judge of their requiring it, as they certainly often do, for their health's sake. The attendants in all asylums have evenings or afternoons of leave in turn, and are seldom refused a day's holiday by the medical officers ; but the officers are prone to confine themselves altogether to the limits of the asylum grounds, if they have to send a written petition every time they wish for a day's change of air and scene. There ought also to be a private gate, of which each officer should have a key, to enable him to escape into the quiet fields occasionally ; for none but those who live in asylums can know how few are the moments in which the resident officers can command relief even to the wearied sense of hearing. Requiring them to be in their houses at a certain hour,— generally an early hour in relation to the customs of their neighbours ; and that every private visitor to them shall write his or her name in a book ; and that the hour of departure of any visitor, if after ten at night, shall be reported to the committee, can merely tend to remind the officers that they are distrusted, and to prevent their either going out as much as their own health of mind and body requires, or receiving the visits of any of their friends, who, naturally enough, object to spend an evening where it is expected that they should hasten away before the clock strikes ten, or have their names paraded before a committee of justices. Habit has reconciled the governing bodies of asylums to regulations which, however applicable to prisons, where security may require them, are as useless, as they must be offensive, to those whose lives are devoted to the care of the suffering and the sick.

For the same reason it is desirable that each officer's household should be independent, having separate servants, and a separate kitchen; and that their salaries should be sufficient to enable them to buy their own provisions. At present, the regulations of asylums vary as regards the table of the officers and all their domestic arrangements, according to the caprice of the committees, and sometimes according to the fancy of the matron or housekeeper. In some an excellent general table is kept; in others, each officer orders his own dinner, and orders what he pleases; in some, fish is forbidden; in some, fowls are prohibited; and committees are said to have been divided on the question of allowing fish-sauces and capers. So, also, as regards the houses of the officers: they are sometimes expensively furnished, sometimes meanly; sometimes their servants occupy good rooms, sometimes cellars and garrets. The permission given to the matrons of asylums to interfere in these latter particulars is incredible and disgraceful. They are now merely alluded to in their connexion with the principle I have already spoken of—that the great object of all the regulations of an asylum should be to direct the greatest possible amount of benevolence and intelligence towards promoting the recovery or amendment and comfort of the patients. For this end, the active services of many healthy minds is the means; and these means can only be secured by promoting the general mental satisfaction and comfort of competent officers, an object which all vexatious, distrustful, and ungenerous regulations cannot but impede.

The medical superintendent himself should deserve the fullest confidence of the governing body, and should possess it. His representations should always be received with respectful attention, and his complaints of neglect of duty, or of departure from his plan of managing the asylum, should be investigated promptly, openly, and with care. His authority cannot be impaired without detriment to the asylum, through every part of which his influence must be continually in operation. The task undertaken by him is one of considerable

physical and mental labour. A daily visit to several hundred
insane persons, each requiring to be accosted so as to do some
good, and to do no harm, is itself singularly exhausting to any
officer whose heart is really in his duty; and the multiplicity
of claims on his attention throughout the day affords his mind
scarcely any intervals of repose. Unavoidable excitements occur, and sometimes he is engaged in scenes of violent agitation, suddenly arising, and where his interference is indispensable. Whatever, therefore, is needlessly done to harass or
depress the mind of an officer engaged in such duty, disquali-
fies him to some extent for his important undertaking; for
vigilantly superintending the whole working of the asylum;
and for consoling, enlivening, animating, and by undisturbed
kindness and calmness ever guiding, supporting, and controlling, more or less directly, the minds of all the rest of the
establishment. It is to him that the whole house must at all
times look for the principles by which everything done in it
is to be regulated. His supposed or his known wishes should
be present to the mind of every officer and every attendant in
every variety of accident, and his character of mind and heart
ever in their view. Indifference on his part must lead to negligence on the part of those who execute his commands; severity exhibited by him must lead to brutality on the part of the
attendants. His steady discouragement of negligence, his
known abhorrence of cruelty, and his real and deep sympathy
with his patients, may be reflected from every humane heart
in the asylum.

His duty comprehends a wide and careful survey of everything that can favorably or unfavorably affect the health of
the mind or the body. He has to regulate the habits, the
character, the very life of his patients. He must be their
physician, their director, and their friend. The whole house,
every great and every trifling arrangement, the disposition of
every officer and servant, should be in perpetual conformity to
his views; so that one uniform idea may animate all to whom
his orders are intrusted, and the result be one uniform plan.

Nothing should be done without his sanction. The manners and language of all who are employed in the asylum should but reflect his; for everything done and everything said in an asylum is remedial or hurtful; and not an order should be given, or a word spoken, except in accordance with the spirit of the director of the whole establishment. By such a system alone can it ever be proved to what extent the cure or the improvement of the insane is practicable.

That he should be a person naturally benevolent is indispensable; and it is extremely desirable that he should possess an almost inexhaustible patience. The qualities to which, of old, much importance was attached—a commanding stature, a stern manner, a fierce look, a loud voice—have become either unnecessary, or positive disqualifications. Threats or reproofs, seconded by these attributes, may terrify the patients, but they loosen the bonds of affection, and generate feelings which will burst forth into expression in the next paroxysm, or revengeful designs, which will wait their time. Even remonstrances, to be successful, must be calm and carefully timed, being, as they are, addressed to the afflicted rather than the faulty. If sickness lays open all the delusions of life, madness often shows all human weaknesses magnified, and they must be viewed with never-failing charity, at no time forgetful that the dispositions so exhibited are impaired and deformed by insanity. The advocates of those gloomy religious views, to which allusion has been made in the commencement of this chapter, are fond of dwelling on what they term the depravity of the insane, and of interpreting the mysterious infliction of madness into the immediate fruits of individual sin. From whatever errors of mankind, ancestral or accumulated, disordered intellect has become so common, imputations thus applied to those afflicted are generally most unjust and untrue. The good feelings of the insane are often disordered, seldom destroyed; control over them and over the propensities is often lost, the will in nowise consenting. Pinel, who well and intimately knew them, says, "I have nowhere met,

except in romances, with fonder husbands, more affectionate
parents, more impassioned lovers, more pure and exalted
patriots, than in the lunatic asylum, during their intervals of
calmness and reason." All my own experience confirms this
valuable testimony; and to persons retaining so much feeling,
all severity must be misplaced.

If the authority of the superintendent is properly maintained, a task which would be irksome and insupportable in
other circumstances, becomes less difficult, and produces solid
gratification. If his labour is considerable, the object of it is
great and good, and the effects are real and appreciable. He
knows that his influence is felt, more or less, by all the patients residing under the roof with him, and he is perpetually
observant of them. In the morning, he notices their state as
regards comfort and cleanliness; at their various occupations,
he sometimes sees and cheers them; at their meal-times, he
ascertains that their food is of proper quantity and quality; he
occasionally joins them in their recreations and exercises; he
meets them at prayers. After the labours of the day, he converses with them, and helps to dissipate the gloom of their
evenings; he often sits awhile by the bedside of the irritable
and desponding, until he has soothed them for the night; he
visits those who are sick, or disturbed, or meditating death, in
the night-hours. He encourages and assists all his attendants, almost at all hours, in their exhausting duties; and he is
always ready to assist them by his advice, or support them by
his presence. By the spirit which, by this devotion of himself, he creates in them, he knows that he multiplies his own
offices and influence an hundredfold.

For the great results of all this, and of all the cares and
attentions which I have attempted to explain, we must look
at the actual condition of well-managed asylums. There we
shall find prevalent a general feeling of trust and confidence on
the part of the patients, and a power in all emergencies which
cannot be in any other way acquired. We shall find a dimi-

nished mortality, an increase in the number of recoveries, and an immense addition made to the happiness and general well-being of all the incurable, including patients of every conceivable variety of sensibility, and possessed of every modification of intelligence and of affection, short of a perfectly sound state of mind, or one free from the certainty of relapse.

I hope my concluding words will be believed, when I say, that if the whole of the system which I have imperfectly endeavoured to sketch be steadily persevered in,—no anger— no severity—no revenge—no deception—no disregard ever shown to the insane,—the resident superintendent will no longer find himself living among the habitually furious, or the incurably gloomy, or the constantly discontented. Calmness will come; hope will revive; satisfaction will prevail. Some unmanageable tempers, some violent or sullen patients, there must always be; but much of the violence, much of the ill-humour, almost all the disposition to meditate mischievous or fatal revenge, or self-destruction, will disappear. Some of the worst habits that beset the poor lunatic will also be got the better of; cleanliness and decency will be maintained or restored; and despair itself will sometimes be found to give place to cheerfulness or secure tranquillity. I could walk through such an asylum as I have described, and point out illustrations of every word in every ward.

Resolved, therefore, to make his asylum a place where everything is regulated with one humane view, and where humanity, if anywhere on earth, shall reign supreme, the resident medical director must be prepared to make a sacrifice of some of the ordinary comforts and conventionalities of life. His duties are peculiar, and apart from common occupations. His society, even, must chiefly consist of his patients; his ambition must solely rest on doing good to them; his happiness on promoting theirs.

None but those who live among the insane can fully know the pleasures which arise from imparting trifling satisfactions to impaired minds; none else can appreciate the reward of seeing reason returning to a mind long deprived of it; none else can fully know the value of diffusing comfort, and all the blessings of orderly life, among those who would either perish without care, or each of whom would, if out of the asylum, be tormented or a tormentor. Constant intercourse and constant kindness can alone obtain their entire confidence; and this confidence is the very keystone of all successful management.

Thus living, and thus occupied, the director will learn to love his people, with all their infirmities, which are their afflictions. The asylum is his world. The patients are his friends; humble, but not without even delicate consideration for others; wayward, but not malignant, except when cruelty exasperates them; capricious, but not ungrateful; distrustful, but to be won by candour and truth; disturbed and grievously afflicted, but not dead to some of the best and purest affections. He will almost regard his patients as his children; their cares and their joys will become his; and, humanly speaking, his whole heart will be given to them.

THE following is a statement of the Cost of Building and Furnishing Twenty-two Asylums, including that of the Land, which in some cases amounts to a large sum. The mean cost for each patient accommodated is £154 2s. 3d., which is probably more than will be found necessary in most future asylums. (From the article LUNATIC ASYLUMS, in the Supplement to the Penny Cyclopædia, published in 1845.) The proportion of land to the number of patients varies considerably. It ought never to be less than ten acres to each hundred patients.

Name of Asylum.	No. of Patients.	Cost. £ s. d.	Cost per Patient. £ s. d.	Land. A. R. P.
Bedford	180	20,500 0 0	113 17 9	9 0 0
Cheshire	152	28,000 0 0	184 4 2	10 3 0
Cornwall	172	18,780 0 0	109 3 8	presented
Dorsetshire	113	14,717 0 0	130 4 9	8 3 0
Gloucester	274	51,360 0 0	187 8 11	24 3 0
Kent	300	64,056 0 0	213 10 5	37 0 0
Lancaster	655	100,695 16 0	153 14 8	45 0 0
Leicester	152	27,630 13 0	181 15 6	8 1 0
Middlesex, (Hanwell)	1,000	202,000 0 0	202 0 0	77 0 0
Norfolk	220	50,000 0 0	227 5 5	4 2 0
Nottingham	200	36,800 0 0	184 0 0	8 0 0
Suffolk	228	32,000 0 0	140 7 7	30 2 0
Surrey	403	85,366 19 1	211 16 7	97 0 0
Yorkshire, West Riding	420	46,846 0 0	111 10 7	40 0 0
Glasgow	350	46,000 0 0	131 8 6	68 0 0 not included in cost
Armagh	134	20,970 4 5	156 9 10	8 0 23
Carlow	180	22,577 16 4	125 8 8	15 0 39
Clonmel	120	16,677 19 3	138 19 7	11 1 14
Connaught	316	27,130 4 6	85 17 1	22 2 28
Londonderry	212	26,282 8 0	123 19 3	12 5 2
Maryborough	170	24,442 19 0	143 15 7	22 2 17
Waterford	127	16,964 12 1	133 11 7	14 2 12

There are in England and Wales 12 county asylums, 5 county and subscription, 11 partly subscription and partly charitable, 1 military, 1 naval, and 142 licensed houses, 14 of which last receive paupers. The hospital of Bethlem, which is exempt from the rules that affect other asylums, is to be added to this number.

Scotland has 8 private asylums, in all of which, we believe, private patients as well as paupers are received; and some are assisted by charitable endowments.

Ireland has 12 public asylums; 10 of these are district asylums for the poor; Cork is locally governed, and Swift's Hospital is founded by charter.

Several new asylums are in progress, both in England and Wales.

With a view to present in a few plain statistical tables the results of treatment in each of the existing public asylums, the writer of this article sent blank forms to each superintendent in the kingdom; in almost every case they have been filled up and returned, and their contents are embodied in the following tables. When information could not be obtained in this manner or from reports, the statistical tables published by the Commissioners in Lunacy have been resorted to; but these only extend to the end of the year 1843, and required much correction, as they are not upon one uniform plan. We may instance the tables furnished by Bethlem and St. Luke's, as omitting many of the particulars desired by the Commissioners. In several asylums no average number of patients is given, and the per-centages of deaths and cures are calculated upon other numbers; in other asylums which have been opened many years, the early records are so incomplete as to be useless. In several asylums, even in some recently opened, the published returns do not contain any distinction of the sexes.

The first table shows the whole number of patients admitted into the 49 public asylums of the United Kingdom to the latest date to which we can obtain information; being 38,537 males, 38,328 females, and 8394 of whom the sex is not specified. Thus the admissions of males exceed those of females by 209, or in the proportion of 1 to ·9945, a scarcely appreciable difference. Of the whole number of insane persons in England and Wales on the 1st January, 1844, according to the Report of the Commissioners, 9862 were males and 11,031 females; thus the females exceed the males in the proportion of 1 to ·894. The greater mortality among men is the cause of this apparent discrepancy.

TABLE I.

Name of Asylum.	Date of. Opening	Date of Return.	Admissions.		
			Male.	Female.	Total.
ENGLAND.					
Bedford . . .	1812	1843	577	524	1,101
Bethlem* . . .	1547	1844	2,658	3,643	6,301
Bristol, St. Peter's Hospital†	1696	,,	265	316	581
Chatham (Military) .	1819	1843	586	22	608
Cheshire . . .	1829	,,	511	386	897
Cornwall . , .	1820	,,	429	329	758
Dorsetshire . . .	1832	1844	202	253	455
Exeter, St. Thomas's Hospital	1801	,,	651	746	1,397
Gloucester . . .	1823	,,	895	804	1,699
Haslar (Naval) . .	1818	,,	807	...	807
Kent	1833	,,	439	325	764
Lancaster . . .	1816	1845	2,384	1,912	4,296
Leicester . . .	1837	1844	284	291	575
Lincoln . . .	1820	,,	577	494	1,071
Liverpool . . .	1792	,,	2,418	1,456	3,874
Middlesex (Hanwell) .	1831	1845	1,399	1,425	2,824
Norfolk . . .	1814	1844	716	794	1,510
Northampton . .	1838	,,	373	368	741
Norwich, Bethel Hospital‡	1713	,,	96	105	201
Nottingham . . .	1812	1845	1,045	808	1,853
Oxford, Warneford Asylum§	1826	1844	...	...	493
St. Luke's . . .	1751	,,	7,130	10,410	17,540
Stafford§ . . .	1818	,,	...	...	3,073
Suffolk . . .	1829	1845	627	620	1,247
Surrey . . .	1841	,,	370	343	713
York§ . . .	1777	,,	...	...	4,032
,, Friends' Retreat .	1796	,,	336	379	715
Yorkshire, West Riding .	1818	1843	1,682	1,657	3,339
WALES.—Pembroke .	1824	,,	16	14	30
SCOTLAND.—Aberdeen .	1821	1845	538	614	1,152
Dumfries (Crichton) .	1839	1844	176	122	298
Dundee . . .	1820	1845	586	505	1,091
Edinburgh‖ . . .		1844	83	79	162
Elgin . . .	1835	,,	49	24	73
Glasgow . . .	1814	1843	1,754	1,421	3,175
Montrose§ . . .	1782	,,	...	...	796
Perth . . .	1827	1845	307	270	577
IRELAND.—Armagh .	1825	,,	800	609	1,409
Belfast . . .	1829	,,	817	776	1,593
Carlow . . .	1832	1844	302	307	609
Clonmel . . .	1835	1845	256	223	479
Connaught . . .	1833	,,	691	472	1,163
Cork . . .	1826	1844	1,739	1,749	3,488
Limerick . . .	1827	1845	906	840	1,746
Londonderry . . .	1829	1843	676	638	1,314
Maryborough . .	1833	1845	296	301	597
Richmond . . .	1830	,,	763	626	1,389
Swift's Hospital¶ .		1844	104	67	171
Waterford . . .	1835	,,	221	261	482

* Only for 24 years.　　† Only for 16 years.　　‡ Only for 6 years.
§ Sexes not distinguished.　　‖ Only for 1 year.　　¶ Only for 6 years.

Name of Asylum.	Discharged cured.		Removed.		Died.		Remain.		Deaths, Cures being 1.	
	M.	F.	M.	F.	M.	F.	M.	F.	M.	F.
England.										
Bedford . . .	217	165	170	185	115	110	75	64	·529	·666
Bethlem . .	1052	1761	1022	1301	220	205	189	197	·209	·116
Bristol . .	117	133	51	71	61	72	36	40	·521	·541
Chatham . .	144	4	156	5	218	7	68	6	1·373	1·5
Cheshire . .	233	197	52	28	138	81	88	80	·592	·411
*Cornwall .	240	225	...	13	113	32	74	79	·470	·142
Dorset . .	87	112	6	13	58	65	51	63	·666	·580
Exeter . .	389	345	157	344	88	35	17	22	·226	·101
Gloucester .	467	457	167	128	121	85	140	134	·259	·186
*Haslar . .	328	...	...	...	356	...	123	...	1·085	...
Kent . .	114	72	35	45	159	71	131	137	1·394	·986
Lancaster .	933	832	152	116	967	641	332	323	1·036	·770
Leicester .	123	135	41	52	45	32	75	72	·365	·237
Lincoln . .	200	189	196	172	124	86	57	47	·620	·455
Liverpool .	1024	548	1083	746	276	144	35	18	·269	·262
Middlesex .	339	337	79	56	563	465	418	567	1·667	1·379
Norfolk . .	308	393	19	21	326	291	63	89	1·058	·740
Northampton	133	153	42	29	74	67	128	123	·556	·437
†Norwich .	43	...	62	...	28	...	68	...	1·581	·581
Nottingham .	450	399	321	232	174	77	100	100	·386	·192
†Oxford . .	246	...	141	...	59	...	47	...	·239	·239
St. Luke's .	2575	4624	3503	4879	959	764	93	143	·373	·165
†Stafford .	1336	...	875	...	612	...	134	116	·458	·458
Suffolk . .	245	278	82	67	188	159	112	116	·763	·571
Surrey . .	57	57	17	9	116	55	181	222	2·071	·964
*††York .	3179	...	...	...	701	...	80	72	·220	·220
„ Friends' Retreat	145	192	67	48	81	85	43	54	·558	·442
Yorkshire, West Riding	686	771	159	218	622	430	213	238	·906	·557

	3	5	...	...	3	3	10	6	1·	·6
WALES.										
Pembroke	3									
SCOTLAND.										
Aberdeen	251	272	85	169	104	87	98	86	·414	·319
†Dumfries	...	...	...	...	...	...	121	91	...	...
Dundee	247	230	129	118	107	64	105	175	·433	·278
Edinburgh	38	52	21	12	11	9	172	11	·289	·173
Elgin	5	7	9	5	3	0	15	...	·6	·000
Glasgow	769	669	556	474	233	130	196	148	·302	·194
†Montrose	324	...	129	...	255	...	47	44	·787	·787
Perth	116	124	60	53	45	29	86	64	·387	·233
IRELAND.										
Armagh	348	282	278	171	109	91	65	65	·313	·322
Belfast	424	428	99	69	152	173	142	106	·358	·404
*Carlow	160	190	...	...	49	39	93	78	·306	·205
Clonmel	154	115	30	18	46	25	62	60	·298	·217
Connaught	239	212	59	36	213	89	180	135	·891	·419
Cork	877	980	288	218	351	330	223	221	·400	·336
Limerick	499	468	69	65	175	129	163	178	·350	·275
Londonderry	313	336	105	85	151	143	107	74	·482	·425
Maryborough	121	156	22	22	68	38	85	85	·561	·243
§Richmond	357	324	169	176	193	117	137	150	·540	·361
Swift's Hospital	46	36	31	16	25	23	73	71	·543	·638
Waterford	98	105	49	69	26	23	48	64	·265	·219
Mean									·624	·458

* Those discharged improved and uncured are included with the cures.   † Sexes not distinguished.

‡ Great doubts exist as to the accuracy of the older books at the York Asylum.

§ There is some mistake here; the admissions are made to amount to 1389, and the cures, deaths, and remaining patients to 1623.

The preceding Table (II) shows the result in the same asylums as to cures and deaths during the same period. This comparative table is recommended by the Commissioners, in addition to the tables showing the per-centage of cures and deaths on the average number.

The cures are taken as 1.

The term " Removed" includes all discharged improved or uncured, or escaped.

This table likewise shows the number remaining in the different public asylums at the latest dates to which we have been able to make up the returns, and which appears to be 5163 males, 5044 females, and 236 of whom the sex is not specified.

The greater number of cures and smaller number of deaths among females must be in a great measure ascribed to their comparative immunity from epilepsy and paralysis, which, when combined with insanity, render recovery very nearly if not quite hopeless. It is also said that women more frequently recover from the acute stage of mania, while men die of exhaustion.

The reverse of this apparent rule is found only in the results of some of the smaller asylums, where the deaths of either sex are few. In those returns where the sexes are not distinguished we have reckoned the proportion as equal.

The tables of per-centage of cures and deaths published by the Commissioners have unfortunately not been compiled upon any fixed plan. All computations, excepting upon the average number of patients in the asylum during the specified year, must be fallacious. The following Table (III) has been made upon that principle. Some asylums do not publish their average number of patients ; others calculate the per-centage of cures and deaths upon the whole number admitted; but this is an entirely delusive method, as these numbers must be continually increasing, while the proportion of patients remaining decreases.

We have, as far as possible, made an average of all the public asylums for ten years past.

TABLE III.—Per-centage of Cures and of Deaths upon the average Number of Patients in the Public Asylums for the Insane in the United Kingdom, for ten years, ending 1845.

Name of Asylum.	Cures.	Deaths.
ENGLAND.		
Bedford	15·88	10·41
Bethlem	40·45	7·30
Bristol	25·05	14·45
Chatham	3·38	10·10
Cheshire	30·09	12·00
Cornwall	13·36	7·91
Dorsetshire	17·95	11·59
Gloucester	30·24	8·92
Haslar	12·95	12·01
Kent	8·29	10·13
Lancaster	17·80	14·94
Leicester	33·90	10·10
Lincoln	19·79	13·33
Liverpool	63·42	16·65
Middlesex (Hanwell)	5·75	8·97
Norfolk	13·10	19·34
Northampton	30·77	13·52
Nottingham	22·29	8·28
Oxford (Warneford Asylum)	22·77	7·52
St. Luke's	44·54	7·86
Stafford	23·17	13·44
Suffolk	16·71	10·49
Surrey	7·63	10·06
York	8·61	6·65
„ Friends' Retreat	8·55	5·24
Yorkshire, West Riding	18·25	14·54
WALES.—Pembroke	8·27	6·22
SCOTLAND.—Aberdeen	16·91	7·58
Dundee	14·70	6·05
Edinburgh	30·61	6·80
Glasgow	48·76	10·02
Perth	13·36	3·99
IRELAND.—Armagh	25·91	8·47
Belfast	28·00	11·35
Carlow	17·62	5·11
Clonmel	21·50	6·80
Connaught	17·74	13·30
Cork	32·69	11·98
Limerick	17·03	6·07
Londonderry	22·17	10·93
Maryborough	13·74	5·93
Richmond	13·08	6·42
Swift's Hospital	9·17	5·41
Waterford	29·60	5·34
Mean	21·26	9·62

The mean number of cures thus appears to be 21·26 per cent., and of deaths 9·62 per cent.; but many asylums depart very widely from this standard. Bethlem, St. Luke's, and Liverpool receive only recent cases; and in the Liverpool institution their probation is very short. The large asylums at Hanwell, Surrey and Lancaster are consequently compelled to receive almost entirely incurables, which accounts for their small number of cures. The large number cured in the Irish asylums may be in some measure accounted for by the peculiar character of their patients. The Irish patients in English asylums usually recover rapidly, the form of disorder being frequently pure excitement, which is soon allayed by quiet, by temperance, and the orderly regulations of an asylum.

Many attempts have been made to obtain a uniform system of keeping statistical tables; at present a different plan is adopted in almost every asylum. A great improvement would be effected if every report, in addition to its information for the current year, contained a condensed statement from the opening of the institution as to admissions, cures, and deaths; and there would be little difficulty in adding the ages, forms of disease, the causes of death, and other tables. Much important information as to the most favorable and unfavorable ages, and the results of immediate and delayed admission, would be easily gained, if a reference to the last report of any asylum were sufficient to show the experience of that institution from its opening in a condensed form. No asylum has yet published any such tables; but in the numerous new asylums which will be built in the course of a few years, nothing could be more easy than to adopt them. The legislature may possibly enforce certain tables; and such a law would be exceedingly desirable, if we could hope that the practical experience of the superintendents of lunatic asylums would be allowed to be of any weight; but if the returns are to be made out according to the fancy of men ignorant of the subject upon which they legislate, the present system, by which every superintendent follows his own discretion, is far preferable.

The following points seem to deserve attention in any plan for uniform registration:

I. Admissions for the current year:
    1. Form of disease.
    2. Causes of disease.
    3. Duration of disease.
    4. Age.
    5. Age when first attacked.
    6. Social state.
    7. Station or occupation.

II. Similar returns for the whole number admitted from the opening of the asylum.

III. Cures for the current year:
1. Form of disease.
2. Causes of disease.
3. Duration of disease.
4. Age.
5. Age when first attacked.
6. Duration of residence.
7. Per-centage upon average number of patients.

IV. Similar returns for the whole number cured.

V. Deaths for the current year:
1. Form of mental disease.
2. Causes of mental disease.
3. Duration of mental disease.
4. Age.
5. Age when first attacked.
6. Duration of residence.
7. Per-centage upon average number of patients.
8. Causes of deaths.

VI. Similar returns for the whole number who have died.

VII. Number discharged uncured, improved, by request of friends, removed by parishes, or escaped, during the current year; distinguishing the reasons for removal, and the duration of residence.

VIII. Similar returns for the whole number removed or escaped.

IX. Patients remaining in the asylum:
1. Form of disease.
2. Duration of disease.
3. Duration of residence.
4. Age.
5. Number probably curable.
6. Number probably incurable.

The registers, to contain all this information, might be of very simple form, far less complicated than those at present in use in several asylums. The sexes should be distinguished in every statement.

Registers should likewise be kept of every instance of restraint, its nature and duration, and of the duration of every seclusion; also of employment and of the value of the work done. Many others might be suggested as useful in various ways, though not strictly necessary for statistical purposes.

7 §

INCURABLE PATIENTS.

The following remarks, arising out of my observation of the improvement in the treatment of incurable cases in the Salpêtrière, were published in the ' British and Foreign Medical Review,' in January, 1845, in a letter to Dr. Forbes, giving an account of some of the French asylums. As they have a direct reference to the question of separating incurable from curable patients, I have thought it might be useful to insert them.

" Nothing does more honour to an asylum than the care and protection it extends to the imbecile and helpless. These unhappy beings may be neglected to a great degree with impunity ; and that in the old asylums they were grievously so, is too well known. Among the objects which gratify me in every visit to Hanwell, none is more entirely satisfactory than the extreme attention paid to the most helpless of the patients, the imbecile, the idiotic, the paralysed, and all who have fallen into the utmost weakness of mind and body ; a state in which they possess no interest for the ordinary spectator, whom they neither alarm by fury nor amaze by eccentricity. Unlike the less heavily afflicted, they can neither appeal to the philanthropy of the visitor nor to the authority of inspectors ; and they would be lost if no compassion were excited by their very wretchedness and squalor, which, however, long pleaded silently and in vain. Among these are not a few whom the physician has traced through successive stages of mental and bodily decay, from the first storm of unreason to the last wreck of sense and intelligence, and who, he knows, can have no friend on this side of the grave if he ceases to be such. It is these abject creatures who have been rescued, by the active benevolence prevailing in asylums, from a state in which it was thought impossible to produce them to decent view. Many a wretch heretofore doomed to lie in hopeless neglect is now daily dressed in clean and warm clothing, and brought out of his bed to sit by the fire or to breathe the fresh and invigorating air. A feeble smile of recognition still passes over the features of these poor declining patients, and not a few of them utter words expressive of their content. They are reduced to the condition of children, and they are treated as children, fed as children, kept clean like children, put into bed like children ; they are only not punished like children ; but are guarded by night and by day from danger, violence, or neglect, until their poor remains of life can be husbanded no longer.

" But for the quality of mercy, in these later times only fallen into their secluded cells, still, among these doomed creatures, in solitude and darkness, and foul smells, the old instruments of restraint would be triumphantly applied as substitutes for all trouble; and wretches still would linger and toss in straw and filth for months and years, through life to death, uncared for and unknown. Those days are past; but their heavy shadow still remains, and obscures humanity still in a kind of defiance of public inspection, and the public exposure of official Reports of the Commissioners of Lunacy. The persevering enmity, too, which has been steadily directed against the reformers of these things, has assumed, year after year, and still assumes so many ingenious shapes, that the friends of the insane must not permit themselves to be lulled into security, or believe that a gradual return to such things is quite beyond possibility. The old arguments against non-restraint, founded on a supposed necessity for other forms of cruelty in the place of restraints, or of a great destruction of clothes and windows, are still continually brought forward by those who first committed themselves by a demonstration of affection for fetters of iron and ligatures and muffs of leather; and the same insinuations are repeated of the insincerity of those who abjure the use of such mechanical methods in the treatment of infirmities and griefs of the mind.

"When I contemplate this, the worst class of incurables, I always think with concern of the disposition apparent in some quarters to make a formal separation, in distinct asylums, of the *curable* and *incurable*. Such propositions are abstractedly pleasing; but the effect ought to be well considered. In the case of many incurables, the manners and habits during a great part of every year are superior to those of the curable, and therefore, not detrimental to curable companions. The separation and transmission to an asylum for incurables would be felt by them as a sentence of eternal imprisonment. As it is, hope, the only blessing left, never dies within them; and some of them recover, after years of affliction, and beyond any ordinary expectation. At once to pronounce many cases incurable which seem so would be to commit many errors; and the asylum for those pronounced curable would always be half filled with cases really not to be cured. The only class, therefore, of the incurable who could safely be severed from the rest of the patients, as mentally dead, would be these poor imbecile, helpless creatures, fallen into fatuity and dementia; and there is much reason to fear that by separating them from a curative asylum they would lose all the benefits which alleviate their unhappy lot. It is quite unnecessary to mix them in wards with more intelligent patients; but it is surely humane to keep them under sufficiently active medical direction in an asylum where it is admitted as a principle that if few cases admit of cure, every case admits of improvement."

SCHOOLS FOR THE INSANE AND THE IDIOTIC AT THE SALPÊTRIÈRE AND
BICÊTRE ASYLUMS, PARIS.

The following passages are also extracted from the account of the
French Asylums in the ' British and Foreign Medical Review :'

" *The Salpêtrière.*—The first asylum which I visited was the Salpêtrière,
a part of which immense institution is appropriated to insane women ; of
whom there were 1600. M. Battelle (Director of the Civil Hospitals,
Hospices civils) accompanied me ; and we found M. Falret, one of the
physicians of the asylum, sitting in the schoolroom, a somewhat small but
comfortable apartment, in which were collected about 100 of the patients,
all perfectly orderly, all neatly dressed, and appearing to take as much
pleasure in the occupations of the school as those who witnessed them.

"To any one accustomed like myself to the daily observation of the insane, the mere appearance of these patients gave eloquent testimony concerning their general good and kind management. Some were engaged
in needlework, which they chose to continue whilst attending to the singing, recitations, and other proceedings of the school. A few only were
absorbed in ideas which no change of place can always relieve. None
appeared to be in any way troubled or fatigued. All were neatly dressed ;
their handkerchiefs and caps presenting the variety and some of the
singularities always seen when the dress of insane females is not regulated
by severe general rules. Above all, almost every one was cheerful, and
regarded the attendants, officers, and visitors without the least indication
of suspicion or dislike. A few of the attendants were sitting among them,
and by their participation in all that was done, contributed to the general
ood effect.

" As the institution of schools in the Hanwell Asylum has been a favorite
object of my ambition, but one in which my hopes have been frustrated,
in consequence of their suppression by an authority which I have no power
of resisting, it was not without the most singular gratification that I be-
held Dr. Falret sitting among his patients, like a father among his children,
encouraging them, assisting them, directing them, and promoting al
kinds of easy and agreeable intellectual exercises that might diversify the
time for the afflicted objects of his care, and, by gentle efforts, lead perhaps, in not a few cases, to the gradual restoration of those powers with
the loss of which all is lost that is worth preserving. The tranquillity, the
consent, the cheerfulness of that little room I shall never forget; and I

trust that the hope such a spectacle inspired of being some day aided in a like attempt among the insane of my own country, will yet be realized before my mortal labours are concluded. At least I trust that the directors of other English asylums will not be discouraged from such an attempt. To have abolished all the horrible instruments of restraint from asylums, and to have substituted the more efficient and beneficial restraint of invariable kindness, is a great work, in which many of our English physicians and directors of asylums have taken part; but they must not imagine that having done this, they have done all. The perfection of their work remains to be undertaken. The end for which this auspicious liberation is but a means must yet be obtained. The troubled brain has been composed, and the heart of the insane tranquillized; it now remains to be seen how far the exercise of the intellect can be restored, and the still more valuable empire of well-ordered affections can be regained. Such aspirations are not the mere results of impressions arising in a scene like that witnessed at the Salpêtrière; they have been strengthened, if not formed, by seeing, day, after day, among the poor objects of our care at Hanwell, the successful efforts of a kind schoolmaster and schoolmistress, with the occasional direction of the chaplain, to teach many very suffering patients to read, to write, to draw, to sing; efforts rewarded by the obvious happiness produced by such occupations, and the perceptible improvement of the mental faculties of some of those engaged in them. When these efforts were no longer permitted, it was among my consolations that Hanwell was not the only asylum in which they had been commenced. The previous labours of MM. Ferrus, Leuret, Voisin, and Falret were not unknown to me; and to witness the happy continuance of those efforts would alone have repaid me for the journey to France.

"The patients at the Salpêtrière have the advantage of a library, and several of them have read parts of the excellent books allowed for their perusal with so much attention as to be able, when requested, to recite them for the amusement of the other patients. Three or four of the women in the schoolroom were called upon in succession by Dr. Falret to do this. Each immediately stood up with much cheerfulness, and distinctly and pleasingly recited a short story or poem. This was done with great correctness; and it seemed as if the patients knew the whole of some long poems, which they went on reciting until stopped, when they sat down with an equal air of content. During the recitation many of the other patients appeared to be attentive hearers. Several of the patients were then invited to join in singing something; and they sung several verses, and in parts, very correctly and agreeably, and apparently without any sane leader. Afterward an Italian patient sung a beautiful air with considerable skill, to the evident satisfaction of her companions.

I saw various specimens of their writing, which were excellent; it was, indeed, with regret that I left this part of the establishment, where, by means of innocent and improving recreations, the patients pass a portion of each day in tranquillity, and, it may even be said, in happiness; and it will be long before I lose the wish to see those cheerful grateful groups again. The school at the Salpêtrière is only a part of what has been done, and what I shall have to describe to you, for the instruction of the insane in Paris.

" This place of careful instruction was but a preface to the whole of the establishment, which I found to be remarkable for its cleanliness, order, and tranquillity. I saw no patients walking about in strait-waistcoats, or muffs, or leg-locks, or handcuffs; and I heard no sounds of raving or fury. At a former visit, in 1828, the restraints and their constant accompaniments had not yet disappeared. In a very recent visit made to them by my son, traces of them were still visible, and attracted his attention by reminding him of our difficulties at Hanwell in 1839. But on the day of my recent visit there was, in fact, not one patient in restraint in the whole asylum.

" *The Bicêtre.*—This large asylum is appropriated to male patients, or rather, as in the case of the Salpêtrière, a portion of the immense hospital is set apart for them, the rest being occupied by elderly or decayed tradespeople and others. About 2000 of these occupy the parts of the building first approached, and the buildings behind these contain 800 or 900 male lunatics.

"The first part of the Bicêtre to which I was conducted was a school exclusively established for the improvement of the idiotic and of the epileptic; and nothing more extraordinary can well be imagined. No fewer than forty of these patients were assembled in a moderate-sized schoolroom, receiving various lessons and performing various evolutions under the direction of a very able schoolmaster, M. Seguin, himself a pupil of the celebrated Itard, and endowed with that enthusiasm respecting his occupation before which difficulties vanish. His pupils had been all taught to sing to music; and the little band of violins and other instruments by which they were accompanied, was formed of the old almsmen of the hospital. But all the *idiotic* part of this remarkable class also sung without any musical accompaniment, and kept excellent time and tune. They sung several compositions, and among others a very pretty song, written for them by M. Battelle, and sung by them on entering the classroom. Both the epileptic and idiotic were taught to write, and their copy-books would have done credit to any writing-school for young persons. Numerous exercises were gone through, of a kind of military character, with perfect correctness and precision. The youngest of the class was a little idiot boy of five years old, and it was interesting to see him following the rest, and imitating their actions, holding out his right arm, left arm, both arms, marching to the right and left, at the word of command, and to the sound of a drum beaten with all the lively skill of a French drummer by another idiot, who was gratified by wearing a demi-military uniform. All these exercises were gone through by a collection of beings offering the smallest degree of intellectual promise, and usually left, in all asylums, in total indolence and apathy. Among them was one youth whose intellectual deficiency was marked in every look, gesture, and feature.

"I think a more particular account of this poor boy's progress deserving of record, as an inducement to the philanthropist to enter on a new field of instruction presenting many difficulties, but yet not unproductive of results. But I must premise that to M. Voisin, one of the physicians of the Bicêtre, the honour seems chiefly if not wholly due of having attracted attention to the various characters of idiots, and their various capacities, with a view to cultivating, with precise views, even the fragmentary faculties existing in them. His work, entitled ' De l'Idiotie chez les Enfants,' abounds with remarks calculated to rescue the most infirm minds from neglect, and to encourage culture in cases before given up to despair. Fourteen years' experience has confirmed the soundness of his opinions; and they have had the sanction of MM. Ferrus, Falret, and Leuret, physicians of the highest distinction in the department of mental disorders. M. Ferrus, who is the President of the Academy of Medicine, and Inspector-General of the Lunatic Asylums of France, was, indeed, the first to occupy himself, so long ago as in 1828, with the condition of idiots at the Bicêtre, of which hospital he was the chief physician. He organized a school for them, caused them to be taught habits of order and industry, and to be instructed in reading, writing, arithmetic, and gymnastic exercises. M. Voisin's first publication on the subject appeared in 1830. The efforts of M. Falret at the Salpêtrière for the instruction of the insane, already spoken of, began in 1831, by the establishment of a school in that institution for idiotic females. Nine years later, MM. Voisin and Leuret, as physicians to the Bicêtre, organized a system of instruction and education on a greater scale. These benevolent and successful efforts deserve to be remembered, as they no doubt prepared the way for the systematic attempt since made at the Bicêtre, where M. Seguin is enabled to apply to practice principles of tuition long recognized as regards the deaf and dumb, but only beginning to be acknowledged as respects those unfortunate beings whose mental faculties are congenitally imperfect in all the various degrees classed under the term idiocy. In this application the master has to educate the muscular system and the sensorial apparatus, as well as the intellectual faculties, or rather the intellectual faculties through them, as a preliminary; doing, in fact, for them by art, by instruction, by rousing imitation, what Nature does for healthier infant organizations. The healthy infant is placed in a world calculated to exercise its senses and to evoke and perfect all its muscular powers, and, to a certain extent, its intellectual faculties. The imperfect or idiotic infant is in the same world, but its senses are, to a great extent, closed to these natural influences, and its powers of muscular motion are incomplete; its intellectual faculties are not evoked by these means, and are even incapable of being fully evoked by any means whatever. The attention is vague, the memory feeble, the imagination futile, comparison is most limited, judgment most imperfect, and all the affections, sentiments, and moral qualities are disordered or perverted. The interesting question is, to what extent can careful and skilful instruction make up for these natural deficiencies; and, as already done for the deaf, the dumb, and the blind, reclaim for these unfinished creatures the powers and privileges of life. The exertions of future philanthropists will answer this question. Improvement must not be looked for beyond what is strictly relative to the imperfect individual in each case; but it would seem to be true of idiots, as of the insane in general, that there is no case incapable of some amendment; that every case may be improved, or cured, up to a certain point,—a principle of great general importance in reference to treatment.

" In the school for idiots and epileptics, at the Bicêtre, a careful register is kept of the psychological condition of each pupil, according to a printed form, for the examination of their instinctive, moral, intellectual, and perceptive state. I was obligingly furnished with a copy of the register relative to the subject of my immediate observations, *Charles Emile*, and also with a copy of the *résumé* or summary of his case, made by M. Voisin himself.

" The age of Charles Emile is fifteen: he was admitted to the school in June, 1843. He is described as being of a nervous and sanguine temperament, and in an almost complete state of idiocy; the faculties which remain being in a state of extraordinary activity, and rendering him dangerous to himself and to others; but still idiotic in his inclinations, sentiments, perceptions, faculties of perception and understanding, and also of his senses, of which some were obtuse, and others too excitable. He was consequently unfit, to use the words of M. Voisin, ' to harmonize with the world without.' As regards his *inclinations*, he was signalized by a voracious, indiscriminate, gluttonous appetite, *un érotisme hideux*, and a blind and terrible instinct of destruction. He was wholly an animal. He was without attachment; overturned everything in his way, but without courage or intent; possessed no tact, intelligence, power of dissimulation, or sense of property; and was awkward to excess. His *moral sentiments* are described as *null*, except the love of approbation, and a noisy instinctive gaiety, independent of the external world. As to his *senses*, his eyes were never fixed, and seemed to act without his will; his taste was depraved; his touch obtuse; his ear recognized sounds, but was not attracted by any sound in particular; and he scarcely seemed to be possessed of the sense of smell. Devouring everything, however disgusting; brutally sensual; passionate,—breaking, tearing, and burning whatever he could lay his hands upon; and if prevented from doing so, pinching, biting, scratching, and tearing himself, until he was covered with blood. He had the particularity of being so attracted by the eyes of his brothers, sisters, and playfellows, as to make the most persevering efforts to push them out with his fingers. He walked very imperfectly, and could neither run, leap, nor exert the act of throwing; sometimes he sprang like a leopard, and his delight was to strike one sonorous body against another. When any attempt was made to associate him with the other patients he would start away with a sharp cry, and then come back to them hastily. M. Voisin's description concludes with these expressions: 'All the faculties of perception in this youth are in a rudimentary state; and if I may venture so to express myself, it is incredibly difficult to draw him out of his individuality, to place him before exterior objects, and to make him take any notice of them. It would not be far from the truth to say, that for him all nature is almost completely veiled.'

"This description not only exemplifies M. Voisin's careful mode of observation, but shows that an example of idiocy less favorable to culture could scarcely have been presented to the instructor. This same poor idiot boy is now docile in his manners, decent in his habits, and capable, though not without some visible effort, of directing his vague senses and wandering attention, so as to have developed his memory, to have acquired a limited instruction concerning various objects, and to have become affectionately conscious of the presence of his instructors and friends. His general appearance is still that of an idiot. His countenance, his mode of walking, all that he does, declare his very limited faculties. Nature has placed limits to the exercise of his powers which no art can remove. But he is redeemed from the constant dominion of the lowest animal propensities; several of his intellectual faculties are cultivated, some have even been called into life, and his better feelings have acquired some objects and some exercise. In such a case as this we are not so much to regard what is merely accomplished for the individual. A great principle is established by it in favour of thousands of defective organizations. After witnessing the general efforts of this school of the most imbecile human beings, and hearing the particulars of Charles Emile's history, it was really affecting to see him come forward when called, and essay to sing a little solo when requested; his attempt at first not being quite successful, but amended by his attention being more roused to it. His copy-book was then shown to me; and his writing was steady, and as good as that of most youths of his station in life. The schoolmaster, who seemed to take great pleasure in the improvement of this poor fellow, then showed us how he had taught Charles to count by means of marbles and small pieces of wood, or marks made on a board, arranged in lines, the first containing an 0, the second 00, the third 000, and so on. Charles was sometimes out in his first calculations, but then made an effort and rectified himself. He distinguished one figure from another, naming their value. Large pieces of strong card, of various shapes, were placed in succession in his hands; and he named the figure of each, as square, triangle, &c., and afterward drew their outlines with chalk on a black board, and, according to the desire of M. Seguin, drew a perpendicular, or horizontal, or oblique line; so effectually attending to what he was doing, that if any line was drawn incorrectly he rubbed it out and began anew. He also wrote several words on the board, and the name of the director of the Bicêtre, (M. Mallon,) without the name being spoken to him.

"This case was altogether the most interesting of those which I saw; but there was one poor idiot standing a great part of the time in a corner, to all appearance the very despair of art; even this poor creature, however, upon being noticed and brought to the table, proved capable of distinguishing the letters of the alphabet. Most of the others had received as much instruction as has been described, and could count, draw lines and figures, write, perform various exercises, and point to different parts of the body, as the head, the eyes, the arms, the feet, &c., when named to them. In all these cases, and pre-eminently in that of Charles Emile, the crowning glory of the attempt is, that whilst the senses, the muscular powers, and the intellect have received some cultivation, the habits have been improved, the propensities regulated, and some play has been given to the affections; so that a wild, ungovernable animal, calculated to excite fear, aversion, or disgust, has been transformed into the likeness and manners of a man. It is difficult to avoid falling into the language of enthusiasm on beholding such an apparent miracle; but the means of its performance are simple, demanding only that rare perseverance without which nothing good or great is ever effected; and suitable space, and local arrangements adapted to the conservation of the health and safety of the pupils; to the establishment of cleanly habits; to presenting them with objects for the exercise of their faculties of sense, motion, and intellect; and to the promotion of good feelings and a cheerful active disposition. The idiot who is capable of playing and amusing himself is already, as M. Seguin observes, somewhat improved.* I can but regret that I had not time to watch the progress of this interesting school from day to day, and to trace the growth of knowledge in the different pupils; as of the first ideas of form and colour, into writing and drawing; the development of articulation and the power of verbal expression; the extension of memory to calculation; the subsidence of gross propensities, and the springing forth and flourishing of virtuous emotions in a soil where, if even under the most favorable circumstances the blossoms and fruits are few, but for philanthropic culture all would be noxious or utterly barren.

"The schools for the insane patients of the Bicêtre, who are neither idiotic nor epileptic, exceed in interest, if possible, those of the Salpêtrière. Male patients are better prepared in general than female patients to derive benefit from such instruction; they are also more attentive and, perhaps, more able to receive various instruction. I have never seen more exquisite penmanship than that of some of the male patients; the drawings of some of them were most beautiful; and I will not attempt to describe the effect of their singing, although I can never lose the impression of it. Here, too, as in the school at the Salpêtrière, the most cheering thing of all was to see the evident comfort and happiness created by the various and not fatiguing occupations of the schools; to witness the satisfaction with which the afflicted, the paralysed, the utterly incurable, exhibited the performances which they yet retained the power to accomplish. If no other end were answered by the formation of schools, they ought to be established as recreative, palliative, remedial even, in every lunatic asylum.

ABOLITION OF PERSONAL COERCION.

The following account of the progressive introduction of what is called the Non-restraint System is extracted (with the permission of the editor of that work) from the article Lunatic Asylums, in the ' Supplement to the Penny Cyclopædia,' already quoted; and it is inserted as containing a brief relation of the principal facts, which are such as to interest every reader.

"No part of the treatment of insanity has of late years excited so much attention as the system adopted in several asylums of totally abolishing

* Hygiène et Education des Idiots. Par Edouard Seguin. Paris, 1843. His larger and more recent work, ' Traitement Moral, Hygiène, et Education des Idiots,' &c. 1846, contains the amplest details of his method.

the use of all instruments of coercion, which has gained the name of the *non-restraint system*. We desire to preserve this name, as many asylums, which still continue to use all the ancient instruments of restraint, endeavour, by professing to practise the 'humane system,' to lead the readers of their reports to suppose that there is no essential alteration made by the discontinuance of the use of those instruments.

" In giving a slight sketch of the progress of this improvement in the mode of treating the insane, we shall consider it as a natural consequence of the progressive amelioration in the management of asylums.

" Until the establishment of Bethlem in 1547, we have little or no records of the provision made for the insane; we can only gather that all who were harmless, and many who were dangerous, supported a miserable existence by wandering and begging; those who could not be permitted to be at large were probably chained in prisons, or in the hands of their friends. Some mention is made of an asylum for insane monks established at Jerusalem in the sixth century, where all the rigours of monastic discipline were embodied in the treatment.

" Even in Bethlem little attention seems to have been paid to the comfort or cure of the patient; the only consideration was the safety of the sane part of the population. The patients were chiefly naked, and chained to the walls, and were exhibited for money, like wild beasts; and it is even said that the keepers were accustomed to allude to every subject most aggravating to the violent patient, that his rage might increase the amusement of the exhibition; while the propensities of the filthy were encouraged, and the voracious idiot was kept without food, that they might appear as more striking objects of wonder to the idle crowd. This shameful practice, by which it appears that an income of 400*l.* per annum was derived by the hospital, was abolished in 1770; but no improvement was made in any other respect in the treatment of the patients.

" The benevolent and courageous Pinel was the first to attempt the restoration of the insane to a position among human beings. The scene of his exertions, which were the first great step of the non-restraint system, was the Bicêtre—hospital for insane men, near Paris. In this frightful prison the universal practice was to load patients with heavy chains, which remained on for the remainder of their lives, and to immure them in dark, unwarmed, and unventilated cells. Pinel determined on at once releasing a large number of patients. The following account of the experiment is extracted from the ' British and Foreign Medical Review :'

" Towards the end of 1792, Pinel, after having many times urged the Government to allow him to unchain the maniacs of the Bicêtre, but in vain, went himself to the authorities, and with much earnestness and warmth advocated the removal of this monstrous abuse. Couthon, a member of the commune, gave way to M. Pinel's arguments, and agreed to meet him at the Bicêtre. Couthon then interrogated those who were chained, but the abuse he received, and the confused sounds of cries, vociferations, and clanking of chains in the filthy and damp cells, made him recoil from Pinel's proposition. 'You may do what you will with them,' said he, 'but I fear you will become their victim.' Pinel instantly commenced his undertaking. There were about fifty whom he considered might without danger to the others be unchained, and he began by releasing twelve, with the sole precaution of having previously prepared the same number of strong waistcoats with long sleeves, which could be tied behind the back, if necessary. The first man on whom the experiment was to be tried was an English captain, whose history no one knew, as he had been in chains forty years. He was thought to be one of the most furious among them; his keepers approached him with caution, as he had in a fit of fury killed one of them on the spot with a blow from his manacles. He was chained more rigorously than any of the others. Pinel entered his cell unattended, and calmly said to him, 'Captain, I will order your chains to be taken off, and give you liberty to walk in the court, if you will promise me to behave well and injure no one.' 'Yes, I promise you,' said the maniac; 'but you are laughing at me; you are all too much afraid of me.' 'I have six men,' answered Pinel, 'ready to enforce my commands, if necessary. Believe me then on my word, I will give you your liberty if you will put on this waistcoat.' He submitted to this willingly, without a word; his chains were removed, and the keepers retired, leaving the door of the cell open. He raised himself many times from the seat, but fell again on it, for he had been in a sitting posture so long that he had lost the use of his legs; in a quarter of an hour he succeeded in maintaining his balance, and with tottering steps came to the door of his dark cell. His first look was at the sky, and he cried out enthusiastically, 'How beautiful!' During the rest of the day he was constantly in motion, walking up and down the staircases, and uttering exclamations of delight. In the evening he returned of his own accord into his cell, where a better bed than he had been accustomed to had been prepared for him, and he slept tranquilly. During the two succeeding years which he spent in the Bicêtre, he had no return of his previous paroxysms, but even rendered himself useful, by exercising a kind of authority over the insane patients, whom he ruled in his own fashion.

" The next unfortunate being whom Pinel visited was a soldier of the French Guards, whose only fault was drunkenness; when once he lost self-command by drink, he became quarrelsome and violent, and the more dangerous from his great bodily strength. From his frequent excesses he had been discharged from the corps, and he had speedily dissipated his scanty means. Disgrace and misery so depressed him that he became insane; in his paroxysms he believed himself a general, and fought those who would not acknowledge his rank. After a furious struggle of this sort, he was brought to the Bicêtre in a state of the greatest excitement. He had now been chained for ten years, and with greater care than the others, from his having frequently broken his chains with his hands only. Once, when he broke loose, he defied all his keepers to enter his cell until they had each passed under his legs; and he compelled eight men to obey this strange command. Pinel, in his previous visits to him, regarded him as a man of original good-nature, but under excitement incessantly kept up by cruel treatment; and he had promised speedily to ameliorate his condition, which promise alone had made him more calm. Now he announced to him that he should be chained no longer, and to prove that he had confidence in him, and believed him to be a man capable of better things, he called upon him to assist in releasing those others who had not reason like himself; and promised, if he conducted himself well, to take him into his own service. The change was sudden and complete. No sooner was he liberated than he became obliging and attentive, following with his eye every motion of Pinel, and executing his orders with as much address as promptness; he spoke kindly and reasonably to the other patients, and during the rest of his life was entirely devoted to his deliverer. ' And I can never hear without emotion,' says Pinel's son, ' the name of this man, who some years after this occurrence shared with me the games of my childhood, and to whom I shall feel always attached.'

" In the next cell were three Prussian soldiers, who had been in chains for many years, but on what account no one knew. They were in general calm and inoffensive, becoming animated only when conversing together in their own language, which was unintelligible to others. They were allowed the only consolation of which they appeared sensible—to live together. The preparations taken to release them alarmed them, as they imagined the keepers were come to inflict new severities; and they opposed them violently when removing their irons. When released they were not willing to leave their prison, and remained in their habitual posture. Either grief or loss of intellect had rendered them indifferent to liberty.

" Near to them was seen an old priest, who was possessed with the idea that he was Christ. His appearance indicated the vanity of his belief: he was grave and solemn; his smile soft, and at the same time severe, repelling all familiarity; his hair was long, and hung on each side of his face, which was pale, intelligent, and resigned. On his being once taunted with a question, that ' if he was Christ he could break his chains,' he solemnly replied, ' Frustra tentaris Dominum tuum.' His whole life was a romance of religious excitement. He undertook on foot pilgrimage to Cologne and Rome; and made a voyage to America for the purpose of converting the Indians: his dominant idea became changed into actual mania, and on his return to France he announced himself as the Saviour. He was taken by the police before the Archbishop of Paris, by whose orders he was confined in the Bicêtre as either impious or insane. His hands and feet were loaded with heavy chains, and during twelve years he bore with exemplary patience this martyrdom and constant sarcasms. Pinel did not attempt to reason with him, but ordered him to be unchained in silence, directing at the same time that every one should imitate the old man's reserve, and never speak to him. This order was rigorously observed, and produced on the patient a more decided effect than either chains or a dungeon; he became humiliated by this unusual isolation, and after hesitating for a long time, gradually introduced himself to the society of the other patients. From this time his notions became more just and sensible, and in less than a year he acknowledged the absurdity of his previous prepossession, and was dismissed from the Bicêtre.

" In the course of a few days, Pinel released fifty-three maniacs from their chains; among them were men of all conditions and countries; workmen, merchants, soldiers, lawyers, &c. The result was beyond his hopes. Tranquillity and harmony succeeded to tumult and disorder, and the whole discipline was marked with a regularity and kindness which had the most favorable effect on the insane themselves, rendering even the most furious more tractable."

" If experience did not always prove that improvements of any kind are slow, and invariably met by opposition, we should be at a loss to account for the fact, that in England, twenty-three years after the liberation of the lunatics at the Bicêtre, a state of things equally bad, if not worse, generally existed. From the evidence given before the Parliamentary Committees in 1815, we gather facts, supported by the evidence of the attendants themselves, almost too horrible to be credible. Every artifice of cruelty seems to have been employed upon those who were already the most unhappy of mankind. The idea seemed to prevail that all the feelings of humanity were extinguished by the visitation of insanity. The keepers were, in all the English madhouses, of the lowest and most brutal character, merely distinguished by their success in controlling the violence of their patients by still greater violence, and by possessing the power of punishment. The account of the inquiry into the management of the York Asylum in 1813, written by the late respected Mr. Gray, gives probably a true picture of the state of the condition of the insane in general. This asylum was opened in 1777, and bore a fair character for organization and management. Upon the establishment of the Retreat, at York, in 1796, a more huanem system than had hitherto been known in England was introduced into its management; and in the description of it by the founder, Mr. Tuke, published in 1813, a recommendation of the milder mode of treatment was given. This was considered, and with some reason, to be an attack upon the management of the York Asylum; and it was followed up by a series of charges brought by Mr. Godfrey Higgins against this latter institution. The horrors ultimately made known would be beyond belief, were they not amply attested, and were it not certain that in some private asylums things are little mended even now. Though the committee of the York Asylum long refused to listen to the charges brought by Mr. Higgins, they could not entirely conceal the facts; and the extent to which frauds of all kinds were carried by the steward assisted much in developing the general state of the house. A committee of inquiry was appointed; and on the day after their deliberations ceased (28th December, 1813), one wing of the asylum was destroyed by fire. There could be no doubt of this being intentionally done; and that it was done to destroy the part of the house most obnoxious to inquiry. How many patients perished is unknown; but at least four were missing. The steward barred the gates to prevent the entrance of those who were willing to assist; and nearly all the officers and attendants were away. The steward entered four patients who were missing as 'died;' but it is far more probable that a larger number was sacrificed. The real number in the house was probably unknown; for either by negligence or design the books had been so irregularly kept, that the number of deaths to July, 1813, actually 365, was entered as 221, and 101 of those dead had been calculated among the cures. The committee refused to adopt the only method of ascertaining the number missing, by requiring from each keeper an account of the patients under his care, from a pretended delicate objection to the divulging of the names of the inmates.

" Mr. Higgins thus sums up the state of the management of the house: —" In the asylum investigations, concealment appears at every step of our progress; 365 have died; the number advertised is 221. A patient disappears, and is never more heard of, and is said to be 'removed.' A patient is killed—his body is hurried away to prevent an inquest. He is cured, but it is by some medicine the composition of which is known only to the doctor. The public cry out that a patient has been neglected; there is a levy *en masse* of respectable governors to quell the disturbance, and to certify that the patient has been treated with *all possible care, attention, and humanity*. A committee of investigation desires to be shown the house: certain cells 'in an extreme state of filth and neglect' are omitted to be pointed out to them. The governors examine the accounts: there are considerable sums of which neither the receipt nor the application appears. They inspect the physician's report: it only aids the concealment. The steward's books are inquired for : in a moment of irritation he selects for the flames such of them as he thought it not advisable to pro. duce. And yet every circumstance of concealment is imputed by some to mere accident; and every attempt to tear off the mask, and exhibit the asylum in its true character, is stigmatized as a libel or an indelicate disclosure !'

" The details which were brought before the committee to exhibit the brutality and profligacy of the keepers need not be repeated; but it is grati- fying to find that Mr. Higgins persevered, notwithstanding all the obloquy. heaped upon him, until a complete change of the officers and of the system was brought about.

" The next asylum of which we shall have occasion to notice the misma. nagement is Bethlem, concerning which we find many particulars in the evidence given before the Parliamentary Committee in 1815.

" The severest restraint and the most cruel neglect seem to have been the almost uniform practice; and it must not be forgotten that this royal hospital, favoured with exemption from all visitation, and from the effects of acts of parliament, has been, until a very recent period, the most deter- mined in resisting the abolition of restraint, in preserving ancient abuses, and in closing its doors against inspection. With such large funds at com- mand, Bethlem ought to be a model where the student of medicine may see every late improvement in the treatment of mental disorder carried into effect, without regard to the economy which has been detrimental to the improvement of many other asylums.

" In 1815 Bethlem appeared to have been going back, rather than improv- ing, for half a century. From the time that the indiscriminate visits of the public had been prohibited, the secrets of the institution were known only to a few. The case of Norris, a patient in Bethlem, which was made public by the parliamentary committee, has often been related ; but it will not be out of place here. William Norris had been an officer in the navy, and was first confined at Bethlem in 1801. In 1803 he is said to have struck Mr. Haslam, the apothecary; and, whether from any real fear of him or as a punishment, a new and most ingenious instrument of torture was in- vented for his confinement. ' A stout iron ring was riveted round his neck, from which a short chain passed to a ring made to slide upwards or downwards on an upright massive iron bar, more than six feet high, in- serted into the wall. Round his body a strong iron bar, about two inches wide, was riveted; on each side the bar was a circular projection, which being fashioned to and inclosing each of his arms, pinioned them close to his sides. The waist bar was secured by two similar bars, which, passing over his shoulders, were riveted to the waist bar both before and behind. The iron ring round his neck was connected to his shoulders by a double

8

link. From each of these bars another chain passed to the ring on the upright iron bar. His right leg was chained to the trough, in which he had remained thus encaged and enchained twelve years. He read books of all kinds, and reasoned quite coherently on the events of the war.' During the whole of this period it was impossible for him, from the nature of the restraint in which he was placed, either to stand quite upright or to lie down at ease. It will be no matter of surprise that he died on the 26th of February, 1815.

" From this time a gradual but very slow improvement in the condition of the insane may be observed. Chains were removed, and leathern restraints of much milder kinds substituted; and more care was given to the warming and clothing of the patients. Some of the largest asylums in England were opened between 1815 and 1825. The introduction of employment by Sir William Ellis at Wakefield, and afterwards at Hanwell, was a great advance in the amount of confidence reposed in patients; employment has since been introduced in almost every asylum, and no serious accident, so far as we are aware, has ever occurred from allowing the use of tools. The credit of declaring the total abolition of mechanical instruments of restraint to be desirable and practicable belongs to Dr. Charlesworth and Mr. Hill, of the Lincoln Lunatic Asylum. The progress of the alteration was given by Mr. Hill in a lecture delivered by him at the Lincoln Mechanics' Institution, 21st June, 1838, and since published with the addition of extracts from the 'Proceedings' of the asylum, and tables showing the gradual disuse of restraint. A reference to a few of these will illustrate this part of the history of the non-restraint system. The Lincoln Asylum was opened on the 26th April, 1820, and was conducted from the first on humane principles, but with all the usual instruments of restraint.

" On the 29th February, 1829, it is reported that a patient has died in the night in consequence of being strapped to the bed in a strait-waistcoat; and an order is consequently given that the use of the strait-waistcoat shall be discontinued, except under the special written order of the physician; and also that every case of restraint shall be entered in a journal, with its nature and duration.

" On the 4th May, in the same year, the ' heaviest pair of iron hobbles,' which were jointed, and weighed 3 lbs. 8 oz., and the ' heaviest pair of iron handcuffs,' which weighed 1 lb. 5 oz., are ordered to be destroyed; five strait-waistcoats are likewise condemned.

"Numerous entries in 1829, 1830, 1831, and 1832, prove the diminished use of coercion. On the 16th July, 1832, is the first order for strong dresses for such patients as tear their clothes. These patients were in all asylums the most subject to continual restraint.

" 21st July, 1834. All the instruments which would confine the fingers were ordered to be destroyed; but manacles for the wrists and leg-locks were retained. March, 1837, the system of restraint was entirely abolished.

Year.	Total Number of Patients in the House.	Total Number of Patients Restrained.	Total Number of Instances of Restraint.	Total Number of Hours passed under Restraint.
1829*	72	39	1727	20,424
1830	92	54	2364	27,113
1831	70	40	1004	10,830
1832	81	55	1401	15,671
1833	87	44	1109	12,003
1834	109	45	647	6,597
1835	108	28	323	2,874
1836	115	12	39	334
1837	130	2	3	28

" Mr. Hill's lecture, which contains much that is exceedingly interesting upon this subject, has the following sentence, which has been the text on which all the controversy on the abolition of restraint has been founded : ' In a properly constructed building, with a sufficient number of suitable attendants, restraint is never necessary, never justifiable, and always injurious, in all cases of lunacy whatever.' This sentence, when published in 1838, was declared, even by those most inclined to the new system, to be too decided, and likely to produce a bad effect ; but fortunately the lapse of eight years has proved its perfect truth, by its adoption as a principle in all the most important asylums in the kingdom. But the upholders of the old system received the announcement of a doctrine so startling as if there were something atrocious in proposing to liberate those who were unfortunate enough to be insane ; and for years after restraint had been actually abolished, the non-restraint system was declared ' utopian' and impracticable ; then declared to be practicable, but not desirable ; and at length, when every other argument has failed, those who have so strenuously opposed it come forward and claim it as their own system, which they have been practising for years, excepting that it is carried a little further.

" Too much stress was laid by Mr. Hill on the necessity for tall and powerful attendants ; and the management of Lincoln laid the early supporters of the non-restraint system open to the charge of using the coercion of fear and of the hands for that of straps and chains. A form of coercion called ' manual detention,' wherein the attendants held violent patients quiet, was actually at one time used at Lincoln ; but it appears to be unknown in the other asylums where restraint is abolished.

" The experience of the Lincoln Asylum has proved every advantage

* From March 16th.

arising from the non-restraint system, notwithstanding divisions among the managers, and direct opposition from some of the medical officers, by whom every kind of unfair evidence was brought forward against the system,' and the cruelties practised by unfit attendants were considered as part of it.

" The next asylum in which restraint was abolished was that of the county of Middlesex at Hanwell. At the time of the appointment of Dr. Conolly to the superintendence of the Hanwell Asylum (June, 1839,) it contained 800 patients; of these about 40 were almost constantly in restraint-chairs, and a number of others wore strait-waistcoats, muffs, leg-locks, &c. In addition to these restraints, which were supposed necessary for the safety of the rest, and of the officers and attendants, more than 100 epileptic patients were fastened by one wrist in bed every night. This was considered a necessary precaution, to prevent the patients from falling out of bed, or from turning on their faces in a fit, and so becoming smothered; which, it is asserted, has sometimes happened. No such case has, however, occurred since the disuse of the hand-strap, which took place in July, 1839.

" We extract from Dr. Conolly's first Report (October, 1839) the following account of the discontinuance of restraint at Hanwell :

" ' The article of treatment in which the resident physician has thought it expedient to depart the most widely from the previous practice of the asylum has been that which relates to the personal *coercion* or forcible *restraint* of the refractory patients. Without any intention of derogating from the high character acquired by the asylum, it appeared to him that the advantage resulting from the degree of restraint permitted and customary in it at the period of his appointment was in no respect proportionable to the frequency of its application; that the objections to the restraint actually employed were very serious; and that it was in fact creative of many outrages and disorders, to repress which its application was commonly deemed indispensable, and consequently directly opposed to the chief design of all treatment, the cure of the disease.'

*   *   *   *   *

" ' By a list of restraints appended to this Report, it will be seen that the daily number in restraint was in July so reduced that there were sometimes only four, and never more than fourteen, in restraint at one time; but that since the middle of August there has not been one patient in restraint on the female side of the house, and since the 21st of September not one on either side.' The 51st Report of the visiting justices, which accompanies this Report, speaks of the new system as requiring an additional number of attendants, and of a superior class to those previously employed.

" In their 52d Report (January, 1840) the visiting justices report the satisfactory results of the new system. In the 53d (April, 1840) they report that 'there has not been a single occurrence to weaken their confidence in the practicable nature of the system;' and also 'that no increased destruction of clothing or other property is occasioned by the personal freedom which the patients enjoy. Indeed, so far as clothing is concerned, the amount of destruction is somewhat lessened, because of the general tranquillity of the patients from the adoption of the new system.'

" In the 54th (July, 1840) and 55th (October, 1840) the justices state their increased confidence in the non-restraint system. This last Report is accompanied by the second Report of Dr. Conolly. During the past year a suicide (by hanging) had taken place, being the only one at Hanwell since the non-restraint system has been introduced. That restraint would not have been very available is proved by the occurrence of the suicide of a female patient in Bethlem, who hung herself in 1840 by the strings of the strait-waistcoat in which she had been confined; and a man has since destroyed himself, also at Bethlem, by working the strait-waistcoat in which he was strapped down in bed so as to produce apoplexy by the pressure of a knot on the neck. The last report of the Lincoln Asylum states that not only have suicides ceased since the system of non-restraint was introduced, but that the tendency to suicide has disappeared. The latest report of Bethlem also contains an admission that restraints increase the tendency to suicide.

" The second division of Dr. Conolly's Report treats entirely of the management of the patients without restraint, and the substitutes for it. The marked improvement in the condition of the epileptic patients is noticed. Seclusion, the most important of the substitutes for restraint is minutely described. This very useful remedial agent is styled by the supporters of the old system 'solitary confinement,' which term is also improperly applied by the Commissioners in their Report. That solitary confinement for days and weeks together was the practice in the days of restraint is certain; for then it was a common practice to strap a patient in bed or in a restraint-chair placed in his bedroom. Any abuse of seclusion so great as this can scarcely now take place. Dr. Conolly says, 'All the substitutes for restraint are, like restraint itself, liable to be abused; but none can be made such instruments of cruelty by abuse. All are also liable to great misrepresentation; and none more so than that which is of all the most useful, the most simple, and the most approved of by the highest medical authorities, namely, seclusion. By seclusion is meant temporary protection of the maniac from the ordinary stimuli acting upon the senses in the refractory wards of a lunatic asylum.'

" In the sixth Report (October, 1844) likewise, Dr. Conolly writes : ' It is to be ascribed to want of opportunities of observation that such a simple exclusion of irritations from an irritable mind—an exclusion not found to be necessary in more than four or five instances in any one day in the year among one thousand patients, and seldom prolonged beyond four or five hours in any of those instances, during which time the patient's state is frequently ascertained by means of the inspection-plate in the door of his room, and all his reasonable wants and wishes are attended to,—should ever have been confounded with the idea of solitary confinement ; the latter in reality comprehending a privation of almost all the stimuli upon which the integrity of intellectual and physical life depends.'

" The room should not be dark ; the shutter which guards the window should therefore be perforated. Care should always be taken that the perforations of the shutters should not be available, as iron bars always are, as ready means of suicide. In the treatment of the insane nothing is trifling ; for upon careful attention to the most minute matters must depend the perfection of management of any asylum;

" The report for 1841 contains many cases which illustrate the benefit of non-restraint. Dr. Conolly also states the result of two years' experience, under sixteen heads, which express that difficulties must be expected in abolishing restraint, from the indolence of attendants accustomed to rely on it, and from the violence at first committed by patients long deprived of freedom of action ; but that if steadily persevered in it will be found to produce greater tranquillity, fewer outrages and accidents, more general cheerfulness, and less obstinacy and malice ; that good effects will be especially observable in patients newly admitted and treated entirely without restraint ; but that complete uniformity of feeling among all the officers, and a sufficient number of humane and vigilant attendants, are indispensable to carry the system to full perfection.

" In this year (1841) a man, aged 82, died in consequence of a kick given by another patient. The injury was not severe, but the weakness and great age of the patient produced a fatal result. The patient who inflicted the injury was subject to epileptic paroxysms ; but was so quiet in the intervals as to be a helper in the wards, and he was actually so engaged at the time of the unfortunate occurrence. This very patient has become tranquil and manageable ; and the ward in which the fatal occurrence took place has become, since the abolition of restraints, one of the quietest in the Hanwell Asylum ; a ward of which the doors are always open, the windows full of flowers, and the airing-court a beautiful garden.

" Dr. Conolly's fourth and fifth Reports (1842 and 1843) contain his confirmed opinion that ' by the abolition of restraint, the general manage- ment of the insane has been freed from many difficulties, and their recovery in various degrees greatly promoted.' The sixth Report (1844) is in a great measure devoted to pointing out the erroneous notions which have been conceived as to the substitutes for restraint, and thus concludes:

"'After five years' experience, I have no hesitation in recording my opinion, that with a well-constituted governing body, animated by philanthropy, directed by intelligence, and acting by means of proper officers, intrusted with a due degree of authority over attendants properly selected and capable of exercising an efficient superintendence over the patients, there is no asylum in the world in which all mechanical restraints may not be abolished, not only with safety, but with incalculable advantage.'

"Here we may consider the subject of non-restraint concluded so far as its practicability is concerned. If no case requiring restraint has occurred in an asylum containing nearly a thousand patients during six years, in which time eighteen hundred cases have been treated, it is unlikely that any more difficult cases can occur elsewhere. It is nowhere insisted that restraint can never be necessary in ill-constructed asylums; and until houses for private patients are constructed for the purpose for which they are used, some restraint will probably be used in many of them. The system introduced at Lincoln, and followed at Hanwell, was very shortly afterwards adopted at Northampton, Lancaster, Gloucester, Stafford, and Glasgow. The new asylum at Glasgow bears on its foundation-stone, laid on the 1st June, 1842, an inscription stating that one of the principles to be adopted in it is that 'of employing no mechanical personal restraint in the treatment of the patients, which had already been abandoned for a considerable time.' The non-restraint system was also introduced at Haslar Hospital, Portsmouth, in 1842, and we gather from the Irish Reports that it has been adopted at Armagh, Londonderry, and Maryborough, and that very little restraint is used at Clonmel and Waterford; and there appears every reason to hope that it will be one of the standing rules in the Irish District asylums that no coercion shall be employed. Dr. Jacob, of Maryborough, expresses his full confidence in the system after an experience of eighteen months. In by far the greater number of asylums which have not yet given in their adherence to non-restraint as a principle, the use of restraint forms an exception to the rule. At Dundee, no restraint has been used for two years; this asylum was one which declared most strongly against the principle of the new system, when first introduced. The reports of Nottingham, Dorset, Montrose, Edinburgh, and Dumfries speak of the advantages of restraint, although the writers abstain from availing themselves of it. On the contrary, the authorities of Bethlem, St. Luke's, Kent, Oxford, and the Retreat at York, profess the non-restraint system, while they practise the reverse.

" The possibility and advantage of the abolition of restraint would seem sufficiently proved by the results reported in all these asylums; but a large number of persons still remain opposed to the new system from various motives. First we must mention the unfair manner in which the subject has been noticed by the Commissioners in Lunacy. A body which had been so long paid to attend to the condition of the insane, and yet who had been proved to allow every evil to remain in the houses under their care, when all others were improving, should have been the last to despise the efforts of others. Their examples of the disadvantages of non-restraint are chiefly adduced from Hanwell, and are most ably answered in a pamphlet by Mr. Serjeant Adams. ·Many of the cases brought forward by them as proving the necessity for restraints, are in fact strong arguments on the other side of the question. The care with which the Commissioners have been selected, until lately, exclusively from persons ignorant of insanity, must be their excuse. The absurdities which they have allowed themselves to believe and to record, would almost induce us to think that they have been wilfully mystified by some of the medical officers of asylums.

" In the Bedford, Chester, Cornwall, Exeter, Leicester, Liverpool, St. Luke's, York, and Pembroke Asylums, coercion still appears to remain in force. The private asylums employ it almost without exception.

" The physicians of the Surrey, Wakefield, and Belfast Asylums have been the most consistent opponents, both in principal and practice, of the non-restraint system.

" With the results before us of the treatment of many thousand patients without restraint, and taking into consideration the facts that in no asylum where the new system has been introduced it has been found necessary to abandon it, that the reports of all these asylums declare their general condition to be improved, that the cures are not decreased, and, which we consider of equal importance, that the comfort of the incurables is greatly increased, we consider ourselves justified in considering that the strait-waistcoat, the coercion-chair, and every kind of strap and instrument of restraint, will shortly disappear like the 'dark house and a whip,' the chains and straw, the starvation, the whirling-chair, and every other means of torture formerly considered a necessary part of the treatment of those who were afflicted with insanity."

(' Report of the Metropolitan Commissioners in Lunacy to the Lord Chancellor,' 1844; ' Report of the Inspectors-General of District, Local, and Private Lunatic Asylums in Ireland,' 1845; ' Returns from each District Lunatic Asylum in Ireland,' 1845; ' Reports' of all ·the principal Asylums in England, Scotland, and Ireland, and information privately supplied by many of the superintendents; Farr 'On the Statistics of English Lunatic Asylums;' 'History of the York Asylum;' Tuke's 'Description of the Retreat near York;' Hill 'On the Management of Lunatic Asylums;' Browne's Lectures delivered before the Managers of the Montrose Lunatic Asylum;' 'Remarks by Mr. Serjeant Adams on the Report of the Metropolitan Commissioners in Lunacy.')

RELIGIOUS SERVICES IN ASYLUMS.

(From the British and Foreign Medical Review.)

The Salpêtrière.—"Although my visit to the Salpêtrière was so long that it would have tired out any less kind guide than M. Battelle, I left it with great reluctance; and having the pleasure of afterward meeting the Abbé Christophe, at M. Falret's, I was glad to have his sanction for attending with him the next day, Sunday, in his visit to the patients. On going into the large church of the Salpêtrière, at eleven o'clock, I found it filled with the numerous pensioners or almswomen of the institution, excepting about two of the portions of the church radiating from the central altar. Notwithstanding all my familiarity with insane people, I at first experienced some difficulty in ascertaining in which of the radiations the patients were seated; so perfectly decorous were they all. At length I recognized the Italian patient, and then others, and placed myself near them, still often doubting whether all those around me were really insane or not; so quiet were they, and so apparently attentive and devout. I stood by them as they moved away at the end of the service, and received many kind nods and smiles of recognition; but there were few of the patients who exhibited much eccentricity of manner. On passing out of the church they walked, four and four, to their own part of the establishment, with the most perfect order and decorum; and their comfortable dress and general appearance were highly gratifying.

" As I differ in opinion from the admirers of mechanical restraints on almost every point of treatment, so I especially differ from them in my estimate of the consolation and advantage of religious instruction or conversation by means of a chaplain, which they naturally enough depreciate. The truth is, that restraint vitiates everything, neutralizes all moral treatment, and reflects disgrace and even ridicule on attempts of any higher kind. It is not so where the patients are treated with uniform kindness

—I would say like children ; but I ought rather to say like human beings. At the Salpêtrière, as at Hanwell, I witnessed the affecting spectacle of a lunatic congregation listening to a sermon. The patients adjourned from the church to the school-room, where the Abbé addressed them in a discourse which lasted about twenty minutes. Everything was done with great simplicity. The patients sat on the benches, the female attendants being scattered among them. The preacher sat at the desk usually occupied by the physician, and I was allowed a chair by his side. A few verses of a hymn were sung by the congregation, accompanied on the piano by a patient. The sermon was very plain and clear, and full of kind and hopeful observations. Most of the patients seemed attentive to it : one or two wept, and others endeavoured to console them. One patient alone became restless, said she heard a voice calling to her, and walked quietly out of the chapel."

[The reader who feels a particular interest in this part of the treatment of the insane, will find it very judiciously spoken of in M. Jacobi's work, already referred to at page 6 ; and very fully and ably in an account published by M. Falret of his visit to the Asylum of Illenau.—*Visite à l'Etablissement d'Aliénés d'Illenau, près Achern, Grand-Duché de Bade.* Paris, 1845. In this admirable little work there is not an opinion on the management of the insane which has not my full concurrence, with one exception ;—the humane and excellent M. Falret being still inclined to lend the sanction of his great authority to the occasional use of restraints, and to designate simple seclusion as *solitary confinement ;* evidently quoting this expression from the Report of the English Commissioners in Lunacy, whose entire misapprehension of the brief and occasional recourse to perfect tranquillity—or seclusion,—as a means of treatment when the brain is actively excited, has misled so many readers, and done such serious prejudice to the progress of the non-restraint system.]

EFFECTS OF THE SEPARATION OF PATIENTS, SUPPOSED TO BE INCURABLE, FROM THE CURABLE PATIENTS.

An instructive illustration of the effects of the arbitrary separation of curable and incurable patients, with a view to provide as cheaply as possible for those supposed to be incapable of cure, has been already afforded in Scotland. One hundred and twenty-three unfortunate lunatics were so quietly transported to the island of Arran, from various parishes on the main land, that the sheriff and other authorities of the district do not seem to have been aware of the importation, until the dangerous appearance of certain wild persons wandering about the island gave them notice of it. The Duke of Hamilton's factor then, happily, applied to Dr. Hutcheson, the physician to the Glasgow Asylum, who devoted eleven days to investigating their condition, and whose benevolent exertions eventually led not only to the removal of these victims of economy, but to the actual cure of some of them, although before abandoned as incurable.

The number of these patients, as reported in May, 1843, was, males 74, females 49. After Dr. Hutcheson had twice visited the island, and sought out all the patients, as well as imperfect returns from parishes, and other arts of concealment, allowed him to do, and before the sheriff could take the necessary steps to compel the different parishes to send their patients to an asylum, their number appears to have been reduced, partly by removals and partly by deaths, to 40 male and 21 female patients. These were sent to the Glasgow Asylum in August, 1843; and, there enjoying every proper advantage, including the care of its excellent physician, 13 of these 61 heretofore condemned and neglected *incurables* recovered, and they are now at large, and supporting themselves; 7 more recovered so far as to be able to live at home; 15 have died; and 26 are yet in the asylum. Twenty poor lunatics, therefore, were by this movement alone restored to social life, and 61 saved from the prolonged neglect and wretchedness which is the inevitable fate of all poor lunatics who, being pronounced incurable, are considered proper objects for a more rigid economy. The honour of this will rest on Dr. Hutcheson's already distinguished name for ever; but the lesson ought not to be lost on persons in authority; for the cupidity of the parishes was still able to ward off humane interference in about half of the cases first reported; and how many are yet lingering in obscure misery no one knows.

The payments made for them appear to have generally varied from three shillings and sixpence a week to nothing; the patients in the latter case exchanging labour for a mere subsistence. Of one of these it is reported that " his clothing was in a wretched state. His sleeping-place was situated between the cow-house and kitchen, opposite the entrance of the hovel; it was seven feet four inches long, eight feet six inches broad, and six feet six inches high. It was damp and ill ventilated. His bed was only five feet three inches long, though he is five feet nine inches in height." In another case a patient was placed in the house of a labourer in abject poverty; living in a house described as " filthy, damp, and ill-conditioned ;" and the only food allowed consisted of " bad potatoes and oat-cake." One poor old woman, formerly in good circumstances, ran away from the wretched hovel in which she was placed under a cruel guardian : " she was brought back, shaken, and beaten with a stick, and shortly afterwards died." Some were deplorably dirty in their habits, and allowed to remain so. Some were sick; but had no physician. " E. R. is in very bad health, and dropsical; notwithstanding which she is lodged in a small closet next the cow-house, five feet ten inches long, four feet two inches broad, with an earthen floor, and without any means of ventilation except the door. Her bed consists of a few boards, a very little filthy straw, and no bed-clothes." Some were violent, and restrained by the rudest methods. Of one woman it is said, " she sleeps in a closet next the cow-house, six feet three inches long, and three feet nine inches broad. Her bed was a box four feet ten inches long, and one foot ten inches broad, containing a little straw and a filthy rug. In this wretched place, without any ventilation, she is confined when more than usually violent." One patient slept in on old cart suspended over the cow-house, to which he ascended by a rude ladder, and where the fowls roosted round him. Various other details are given by Dr. Hutcheson, and generally of a revolting kind. I have myself not the smallest doubt that there are many insane paupers now in England whose treatment is not better; and if the commissioners or the magistracy disregard them, or give the slightest encouragement to their being disregarded as incurables, their condition will be long before it is improved. On the private feelings of neighbours, or even of relatives, no reliance can be placed. The condition of the 61 patients rescued from the exile of the island of Arran by Dr. Hutcheson, would probably never have been reported to him if the dangerous violence of some of them had not alarmed the inhabitants. Their filth, their starvation, their various sufferings from brutal guardians, do not seem to have awakened any sympathy; but as dangerous persons " on the Duke of Hamilton's property in Arran," they excited the attention which led to relief.

It would be unjust to attach to the parish officers all the odium of this transportation of lunatics to Arran. Among the persons confided to the care of the poor inhabitants was the sister of a banker, of imbecile mind from infancy; and of her the Report says, " Twenty pounds a year are paid as board; but though her friends are wealthy, they wish to reduce it. We found her milking cows, and in the garb of the lowest menial." It is on the public, therefore, and on well-informed public authorities, that the fate of the poor lunatic altogether depends. (*Poor Law Inquiry, Scotland, Appendix, Part III.*)

PLANS OF ASYLUMS.

Two of the following plans are appended as being in almost every material point accordant with the principles maintained in the preceding chapters; and containing perhaps every possible provision for the health, proper treatment, and recovery of the insane. The third plan shows some of the modifications rendered necessary in warmer climates.

PLAN OF THE DERBY ASYLUM.

The first in order is the ground plan of that of Messrs. Paterson and Duesbury for the Lunatic Asylum at Derby, to which particular reference has been made in Chapter I. The plan is for 360 patients; and provides for rather less than two thirds of single rooms. In this plan I found, for the first time, that arrangement of the linear part of the building (A and B) by which each gallery has the advantage of a cheerful window at the end. The extended front, the wings at right angles, the disposition of the private rooms, chapel, kitchen, offices, workshops, baths, airing-courts, &c., constitute some of its recommendations; and all the minor arrangments, as regards staircases, water-closets, supply of water, drainage, warming and ventilating, &c., appear to have been very carefully considered.

The references A, A, B, B, C, C, *a, a, b, b, c, c,* show the facilities afforded by an asylum of this form for the classification of patients within doors and without. The compartments for meals, 1, 1, 1, 1, 1, 1, and the bay-windows in each gallery, half way from each end, are new, I think, in plans for asylums, and more favorable, in my opinion, to the constant superintendence of the patients than the old day-rooms. Washing-rooms for the patients, 3, 3, 3, 3, 3, 3, are also novelties in the original plan of an asylum; and much to be commended. The corridor of communication, 8, 8, has many conveniences, although open, perhaps, to objections already spoken of. The visitor's rooms, 13, 13, are also the reception-rooms of patients on admission; and from these they can be taken through the corridor to any particular ward, without traversing others. This plan merely shows the ground-floor. The situation of the chapel and school-room, or music-room, is in the next story, above the kitchen and offices.

PLAN OF AN ASYLUM FOR HALIFAX, NOVA-SCOTIA.

This plan is prepared by Mr. Harris, the resident engineer at the Asylum at Hanwell; and although evidently bearing a resemblance to the general outline of the plan for the Derby Asylum, presents several modifications resulting from long experience acquired as an officer resident in an asylum.

The central part of the building, the offices behind it, and the small advancing wings, form an asylum for 200 patients; the additional wings (1, 1, 2, 2, 3, 3, 4, 4) would render the whole building capable of containing 444 patients. Its length, completed, would be 615 feet; and it would contain 232 single bedrooms.

A certain economy of frontage is obtained in this plan, without having recourse to the objectionable arrangement of sleeping-rooms on both sides of the galleries. Equidistant from both of the well-lighted ends of each gallery, a dormitory and two attendants' rooms, or, in the refractory wards, six single rooms, are placed on the side of the gallery opposite the general range of sleeping-rooms. This affords much additional accommodation for patients, and is thought to render it easier to preserve an equal temperature in the galleries both in winter and summer.

The situation of the visitors' rooms, which are also the reception rooms of new patients (k, k) is such that the patients can go from or be brought to them direct from any of the galleries, without passing through wards to which they do not belong.

A small third story is added over the two small advancing wings; and the portion of it behind the infirmaries contains large rooms, capable of subdivision, for schools or workrooms.

I entertain great objections to third stories in asylums, for any purposes whatever; but taking the whole of this plan together, its conveniences will be very evident on a minute examination.

PLAN OF THE ASYLUM AT KINGSTON, JAMAICA.

The plan of this Asylum, also designed by Mr. Harris, has little resemblance to those described as suitable to temperate climates. Protection from the burning sun, means of ventilation without the admission of the heated air, or even of the glowing daylight, are indispensable requisites for an asylum within the tropics.

This asylum is to contain about 250 patients. In the advanced front building are the apartments of the governor, and accommodation for about 26 patients of the upper class. The offices form a long retiring line behind this building, having on each side of it three distinct buildings parallel with it, but separated from it and from each other by airing-courts. Each of these six parallel buildings constitutes a ward, containing a gallery, and bedrooms for about 37 patients; the rooms being arranged on both sides of the gallery. Three of these wards are for male, and three for female patients. The Bird's-eye View, which Mr. Harris has obligingly appended to the plan, shows the arrangement of these buildings very clearly; and the spacious verandas, about ten feet in width, with which each, as well as the front building, is provided. These verandas have open railings at the ends. The site chosen is near the sea, of which, and of the shipping in Kingston Harbour, the ha-ha fences permit views to the patients. There is a small infirmary on each side of the asylum; detached from the other buildings, but easy of access. Provision for the admission of cool air is made in the basement story: the whole of which, having floors of concrete to prevent the ascent of damp, forms a vast air-chamber; the air being admitted through gratings in the external walls, and passing up flues into the wards; from whence it can be drawn through large funnels with caps made to open and close as required.

The adoption of this plan by the council of Jamaica, is a sufficient proof of its being considered suitable to the climate; and it is gratifying to know that it is the wish of the Commissioners appointed to erect it, that it should possess all the conveniences of an European establishment. This is a great step in the improvement of Colonial Asylums. It is to be regretted that an excellent plan by Mr. Harris, for an asylum at Colombo, in Ceylon, appears to have been abandoned by the council of that important island; to the asylum of which Dr. James Davey, one of the medical officers of the Hanwell Asylum, was appointed in 1844. The officers attached to the asylums on the continent of India are also apparently anxious to improve their condition: but it must always be remembered that the want of a properly constructed building, erected especially for the insane, constitutes an obstacle, almost insuperable, to the introduction of improvements of any kind.

C. AND J. ADLARD, PRINTERS, BARTHOLOMEW CLOSE.

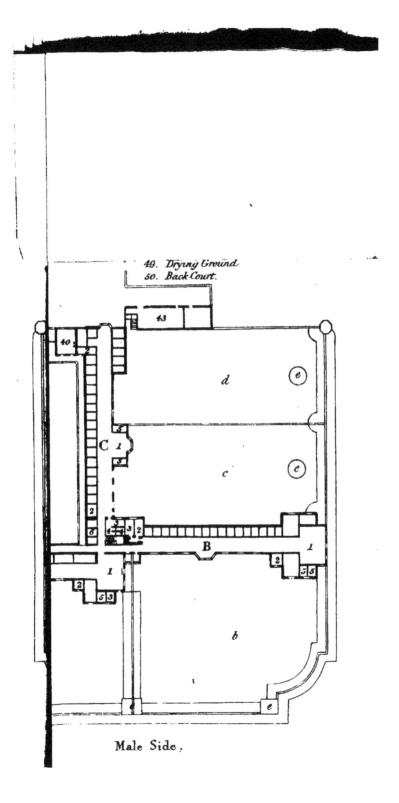

49. Drying Ground
50. Back Court.

43

40

d   e

C 1

c   e

2

6   4   3   2

B

1

1

2   5   5

2

5   3

b

e

Male Side.

J. HARRIS, ARCH⁺

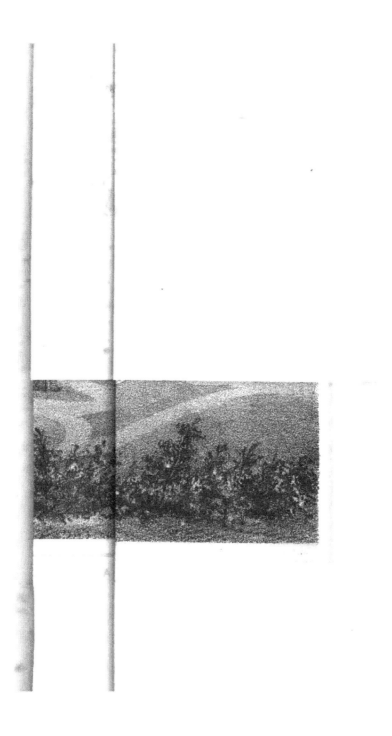

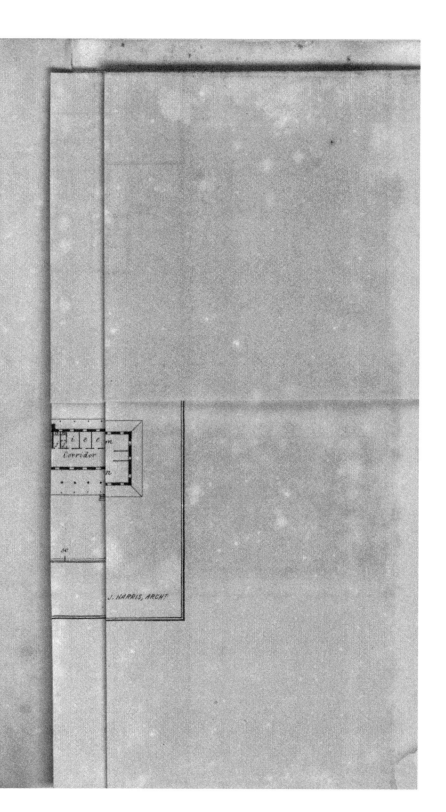

Corridor

J. HARRIS, ARCH.T